Respiratory Physiology

—the essentials
4th edition

Respiratory Physiology

—the essentials
4th edition

John B. West, MD, PhD, DSc

Professor of Medicine and Physiology
University of California, San Diego
School of Medicine
La Jolla, California

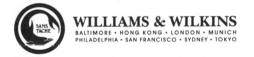

WILLIAMS & WILKINS
BALTIMORE • HONG KONG • LONDON • MUNICH
PHILADELPHIA • SAN FRANCISCO • SYDNEY • TOKYO

Editor: Timothy S. Satterfield
Associate Editor: Linda Napora
Copy Editor: Thomas Lehr
Design: Frank Daniel
Illustration Planning: Wayne Hubbel
Production: Charles E. Zeller

Printed in the United States of America

First edition, 1974
Second edition, 1979
Third edition, 1985

French translation, 1975, 1986; Spanish translation, 1976; Iranian translation, 1976; Portuguese translation, 1977; Italian translation, 1978; Chinese translation, 1979; Japanese translation, 1981; Dutch translation, 1981; Bahasa Malaysia translation, 1984; Russian translation, 1988; Greek translation, 1988

Library of Congress Cataloging-in-Publication Data

West, John B. (John Burnard)
  Respiratory physiology—the essentials / John B. West.—4th ed.
    p.   cm.
  Companion v. to: Pulmonary pathophysiology—the essentials / John B. West. 3rd ed. c1987.
  Bibliography: p.
  Includes index.
  ISBN 0-683-08942-0
  1. Respiration. I. West, John B. (John Burnard). Pulmonary pathophysiology—the essentials. 3rd ed. II. Title.
  [DNLM: 1. Respiration.   WF 102 W518r]
QP121.W43 1990
612'.2—dc19
DNLM/DLC
for Library of Congress   89-5394
                                                                    CIP

91 92 93
4   5   6   7   8   9   10

To P.H.W.

Preface to the Fourth Edition

Several sections of the book have been updated, including those devoted to the pulmonary circulation, metabolism, ventilation-perfusion relationships, blood-gas transport, mechanics, and the control of ventilation. However, the temptation to enlarge the book has been resisted. Areas such as pulmonary edema and the lung's defense system, which lie on the borderland between physiology and pathophysiology, are briefly dealt with here, but more extensive accounts can be found in the companion volume, JB West: *Pulmonary Pathophysiology—the essentials,* 3rd edition, Baltimore, Williams & Wilkins, 1987. Recent research has resulted in a blurring of the distinction between respiratory physiology and related topics such as pulmonary cell biology, immunology, and pharmacology. While these topics are alluded to in various places, the book continues to concentrate on the essentials of respiratory physiology. Sets of audio tapes with slides are available to supplement both this book and the companion volume, *Pulmonary Pathophysiology— the essentials.* These can be obtained from Audio Visual Medical Marketing, Inc., 235 Park Avenue South, New York, NY 10003.

Contents

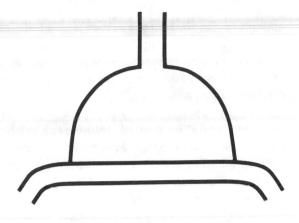

chapter **1**

Structure and Function

*how the architecture of the
lung subserves its function*

The lung is for gas exchange. Its prime function is to allow oxygen
to move from the air into the venous blood and carbon dioxide to
move out. The lung does other jobs too. It metabolizes some compounds, filters toxic materials from the circulation, and acts as a
reservoir for blood. But its cardinal function is to exchange gas, and
we shall therefore begin at the blood-gas interface where the gas
exchange occurs.

BLOOD-GAS INTERFACE

Oxygen and carbon dioxide move between air and blood by <u>simple</u>
<u>diffusion,</u> that is, from an area of high to low partial pressure,* much

---

*The partial pressure of a gas is found by multiplying its concentration by the total
pressure. For example, dry air has 20.93% O_2. Its partial pressure (P_{O_2}) at sea level
(barometric pressure 760 mm Hg) is 20.93/100 × 760 = 159 mm Hg. When air is

as water runs downhill. Fick's law of diffusion states that the amount of gas that moves across a sheet of tissue is proportional to the area of the sheet but inversely proportional to its thickness. The blood-gas barrier is exceedingly thin (Figure 1.1) and has an area of between 50 and 100 square meters. It is therefore well suited to its function of gas exchange.

How is it possible to obtain such a prodigious surface area for diffusion inside the limited thoracic cavity? By wrapping the small blood vessels (capillaries) around an enormous number of small air sacs called *alveoli* (Figure 1.2). There are about 300 million alveoli in the human lung, each about ⅓ mm in diameter. If they were spheres,† their total surface area would be 85 square meters, but their volume only 4 liters. By contrast, a single sphere of this volume would have an internal surface area of only ¹⁄₁₀₀ square meter. Thus the lung generates this large diffusion area by being divided into myriads of units.

Gas is brought to one side of the blood-gas interface by *airways* and blood to the other side by *blood vessels*.

AIRWAYS AND AIR FLOW

The airways consist of a series of branching tubes which become narrower, shorter, and more numerous as they penetrate deeper into the lung (Figure 1.3). The *trachea* divides into right and left main bronchi, which in turn divide into lobar, then segmental bronchi. This process continues down to the *terminal bronchioles,* which are the smallest airways without alveoli. All these bronchi make up the *conducting airways*. Their function is to lead inspired air to the gas exchanging regions of the lung (Figure 1.4). Since the conducting airways contain no alveoli and therefore themselves take no part in gas exchange, they constitute the *anatomic dead space*. Its volume is about 150 ml.

The terminal bronchioles divide into *respiratory bronchioles,* which have occasional alveoli budding from their walls, Finally, we

---

inhaled into the upper airways, it is warmed and moistened, and the water vapor pressure is then 47 mm Hg, so that the total dry gas pressure is only $760 - 47 = 713$ mm Hg. The P_{O_2} of inspired air is therefore $20.93/100 \times 713 = 149$ mm Hg. A liquid exposed to a gas until equilibration takes place has the same partial pressure as the gas. For a more complete description of the gas laws, see the Appendix.

† The alveoli are not spherical but polyhedral. Nor is the whole of their surface available for diffusion (see Figure 1.1). These numbers are therefore only approximate.

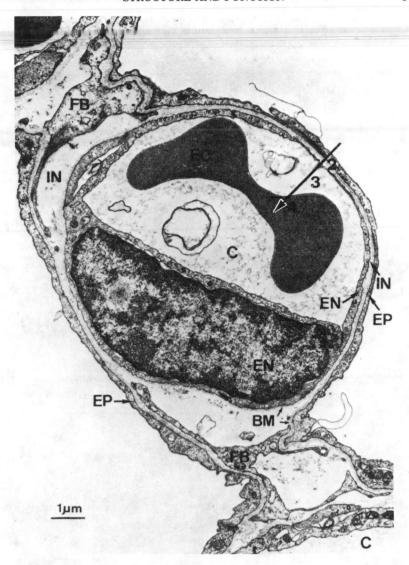

Figure 1.1.   Electron micrograph showing a pulmonary capillary (*C*) in the alveolar wall. Note the extremely thin blood-gas barrier of less than 0.5 micron in some places. The *large arrow* indicates the diffusion path from alveolar gas to the interior of the erythrocyte and includes the layer of surfactant (not shown in the preparation), alveolar epithelium (*EP*), interstitium (*IN*), capillary endothelium (*EN*), and plasma. Parts of structural cells called fibroblasts (*FB*), basement membrane (*BM*), and a nucleus of an endothelial cell are also seen. (From ER Weibel: *Respir Physiol* 11:54, 1970.)

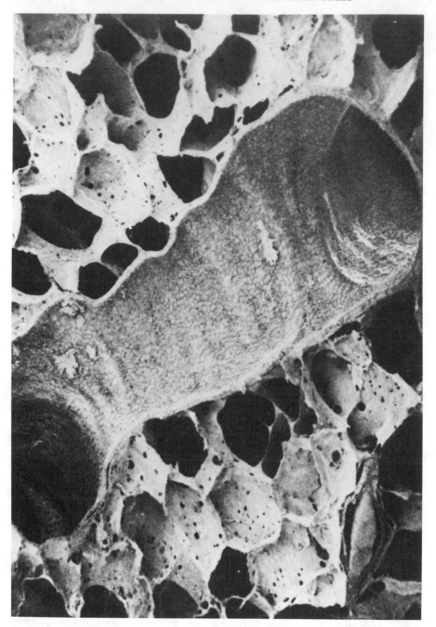

Figure 1.2. Section of lung showing many alveoli and a small bronchiole. The pulmonary capillaries run in the walls of the alveoli (Figure 1.1). The holes in the alveolar walls are the pores of Kohn. (Scanning electron micrograph by JA Nowell and WS Tyler.)

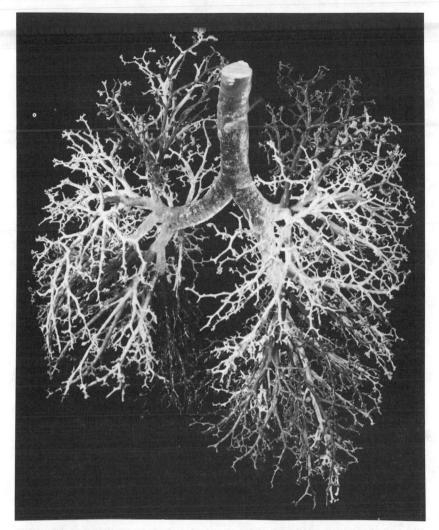

Figure 1.3. Cast of the airways of a human lung. The alveoli have been pruned away, but the conducting airways from the trachea to the terminal bronchioles can be seen.

come to the *alveolar ducts,* which are completely lined with alveoli. This alveolated region of the lung where the gas exchange occurs is known as the *respiratory zone.* The portion of lung distal to a terminal bronchiole forms an anatomical unit called the *acinus* or *lobule.* The distance from the terminal bronchiole to the most distal alveolus is only a few mm, but the respiratory zone makes up most of the lung, its volume being about 3000 ml.

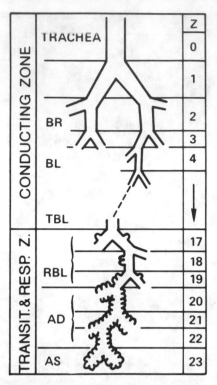

Figure 1.4. Idealization of the human airways according to Weibel. Note that the first 16 generations (*Z*) make up the conducting airways and the last 7 the respiratory zone (or the transitional and respiratory zone). *BR*, bronchus; *BL*, bronchiole; *TBL*, terminal bronchiole; *RBL*, respiratory bronchiole; *AD*, alveolar duct; *AS*, alveolar sac. (From ER Weibel: *Morphometry of the Human Lung.* Berlin, Springer-Verlag, 1963, p 111.)

During inspiration, the volume of the thoracic cavity increases and air is drawn into the lung. The increase in volume is brought about partly by contraction of the diaphragm, which causes it to descend, and partly by the action of the intercostal muscles, which raise the ribs, thus increasing the cross-sectional area of the thorax. Inspired air flows down to about the terminal bronchioles by bulk flow, like water through a hose. Beyond that point, the combined cross-sectional area of the airways is so enormous because of the large number of branches (Figure 1.5) that the forward velocity of the gas becomes very small. Diffusion of gas within the airways then takes over as the dominant mechanism of ventilation in the respiratory zone. The rate of diffusion of gas molecules within the airways

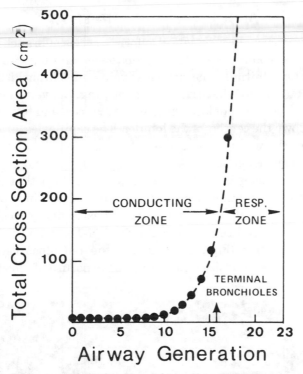

Figure 1.5. Diagram to show the extremely rapid increase in total cross-sectional area of the airways in the respiratory zone (compare Figure 1.4). As a result, the forward velocity of the gas during inspiration becomes very small in the region of the respiratory bronchioles, and gaseous diffusion becomes the chief mode of ventilation.

is so rapid, and the distances to be covered are so short, that differences in concentration within the acinus are virtually abolished within a second. However, because the velocity of gas falls rapidly in the region of the terminal bronchioles, inhaled dust frequently settles out there.

The lung is elastic and returns passively to its preinspiratory volume during resting breathing. It is remarkably easy to distend. For example, a normal breath of about 500 ml requires a distending pressure of less than 3 cm water. By contrast, a child's balloon may need a pressure of 30 cm water for the same change in volume.

The pressure required to move gas through the airways is also very small. During normal inspiration, an air flow rate of 1 liter/sec requires a pressure drop along the airways of less than 2 cm water. Compare a smoker's pipe which needs a pressure of about 500 cm water for the same flow rate.

BLOOD VESSELS AND FLOW

The pulmonary blood vessels also form a series of branching tubes from the *pulmonary artery* to the *capillaries* and back to the *pulmonary veins*. Initially the arteries, veins, and bronchi run close together, but toward the periphery of the lung, the veins move away to pass between the lobules, whereas the arteries and bronchi travel together down the centers of the lobules. The capillaries form a dense network in the walls of the alveoli (Figure 1.6). The diameter of a capillary segment is about 10 microns, just large enough for a red blood cell. The lengths of the segments are so short that the dense network forms an almost continuous sheet of blood in the alveolar wall, a very efficient arrangement for gas exchange. Alveolar walls are not often seen face on, as in Figure 1.6. The usual thin microscopic cross-section (Figure 1.7) shows the red blood cells in the capillaries and emphasizes the enormous exposure of blood to aveo-

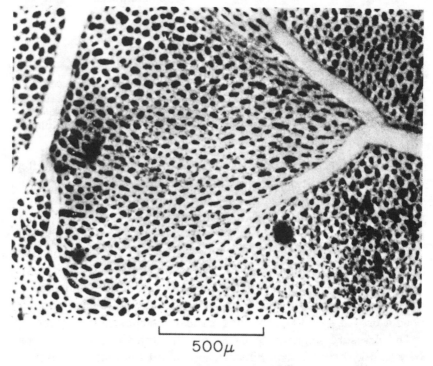

500μ

Figure 1.6. View of an alveolar wall (in the frog) showing the dense network of capillaries. A small artery (*left*) and vein (*right*) can also be seen. The individual capillary segments are so short that the blood forms an almost continuous sheet. (From JE Maloney and BL Castle: *Respir Physiol* 7:150, 1969.)

lar gas, with only the thin blood-gas barrier intervening (compare Figure 1.1).

The pulmonary artery receives the whole output of the right heart, but the resistance of the pulmonary circuit is astonishingly small. A mean pulmonary arterial pressure of only about 20 cm water (about 15 mm Hg) is required for a flow of 6 liters/min. (The same flow through a soda straw needs 120 cm water.)

Each red blood cell spends about ¾ sec in the capillary network and during this time probably traverses two or three alveoli. So efficient is the anatomy for gas exchange that this brief time is sufficient for virtually complete equilibration of oxygen and carbon dioxide between alveolar gas and capillary blood.

The lung has an additional blood system, the bronchial circulation, which supplies the conducting airways down to about the terminal bronchioles. Most of this blood is carried away from the lung via the pulmonary veins. The flow through the bronchial circulation is a mere fraction of that through the pulmonary circulation, and the

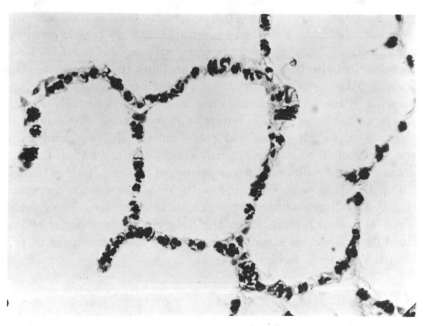

Figure 1.7. Microscopic section of dog lung showing capillaries in the alveolar walls. The blood-gas barrier is so thin that it cannot be identified here (compare Figure 1.1). This section was prepared from lung which was rapidly frozen while being perfused. (From JB Glazier, JMB Hughes, JE Maloney, and JB West: *J Appl Physiol* 26:65, 1969.)

lung can function fairly well without it, for example, following lung transplantation.

To conclude this brief account of the functional anatomy of the lung, let us glance at two special problems that the lung has overcome.

STABILITY OF ALVEOLI

The lung can be regarded as a collection of 300 million bubbles each 0.3 mm in diameter. Such a structure is inherently unstable. Because of the surface tension of the liquid lining the alveoli, relatively large forces develop which tend to collapse alveoli. Fortunately some of the cells lining the alveoli secrete a material called *surfactant* which dramatically lowers the surface tension of the alveolar lining layer (see Chapter 7). As a consequence, the stability of the alveoli is enormously increased, although collapse of small air spaces is always a potential problem and frequently occurs in disease.

REMOVAL OF INHALED PARTICLES

With its surface area of 50–100 square meters, the lung presents the largest surface of the body to an increasingly hostile environment. Various mechanisms for dealing with inhaled particles have been developed (see Chapter 9). Large particles are filtered out in the nose. Smaller particles which deposit in the conducting airways are removed by a moving staircase of mucus which continually sweeps debris up to the epiglottis, where it is swallowed. The mucus is secreted by mucous glands and goblet cells in the bronchial walls and is propelled by millions of tiny cilia which move rhythmically under normal conditions but are paralyzed by some inhaled toxins.

The alveoli have no cilia, and particles which deposit there are engulfed by large wandering cells called macrophages. The foreign material is then removed from the lung via the lymphatics or the blood flow. Blood cells such as leukocytes also participate in the defense reaction to foreign material.

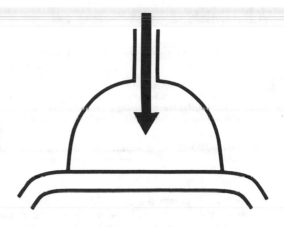

chapter 2

Ventilation

how gas gets to the alveoli

The next three chapters are concerned with how inspired air gets to the alveoli, how gases cross the blood-gas interface, and how they are removed from the lung by the blood. These functions are carried out by ventilation, diffusion, and blood flow, respectively.

Figure 2.1 is a highly simplified diagram of a lung. The various bronchi which make up the conducting airways (Figures 1.3 and 1.4) are now represented by a single tube labeled anatomic dead space. This leads into the gas exchanging region of the lung which is bounded by the blood-gas interface and the pulmonary capillary blood. With each inspiration, about 500 ml of air enters the lung (*tidal volume*). Note how small a proportion of the total lung volume is represented by the anatomic dead space. Also note the very small volume of capillary blood, compared with that of alveolar gas (compare Figure 1.7).

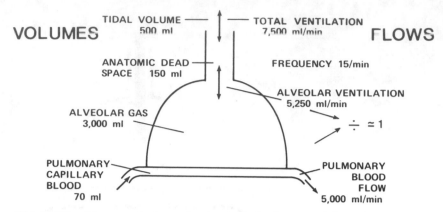

VOLUMES

TIDAL VOLUME ——
500 ml

ANATOMIC DEAD
SPACE   150 ml

ALVEOLAR GAS
3,000 ml

PULMONARY
CAPILLARY
BLOOD
70 ml

FLOWS

TOTAL VENTILATION
7,500 ml/min

FREQUENCY 15/min

ALVEOLAR VENTILATION
5,250 ml/min

$\div \approx 1$

PULMONARY
BLOOD
FLOW
5,000 ml/min

Figure 2.1. Diagram of a lung showing typical volumes and flows. There is considerable variation around these values. (Modified from JB West: *Ventilation/Blood Flow and Gas Exchange,* ed 4. Oxford, Blackwell, 1985, p 3.)

LUNG VOLUMES

Before looking at the movement of gas into the lung, a brief glance at the static volumes of the lung is helpful. Some of these can be measured with a spirometer (Figure 2.2). During exhalation, the bell goes up and the pen down, marking a moving chart. First, normal breathing can be seen (*tidal volume*). Next the subject took a maximal inspiration and followed this by a maximal expiration. The exhaled volume is called the *vital capacity*. However, some gas remained in the lung after a maximal expiration; this is the *residual volume*. The volume of gas in the lung after a normal expiration is the *functional residual capacity*.

Neither the functional residual capacity nor the residual volume can be measured with a simple spirometer. However, a gas dilution technique can be used as shown in Figure 2.3. The subject is connected to a spirometer containing a known concentration of helium, which is virtually insoluble in blood. After some breaths, the helium concentrations in the spirometer and lung become the same. Since no helium has been lost, the amount of helium present before equilibration (concentration × volume) is $C_1 \times V_1$ and equals the amount after equilibration, $C_2 \times (V_1 + V_2)$. From this, $V_2 = V_1(C_1 - C_2)/C_2$. In practice, oxygen is added to the spirometer during equilibration to make up for that consumed by the subject, and also carbon dioxide is absorbed.

Another way of measuring the functional residual capacity (FRC)

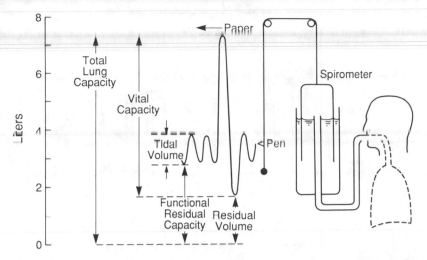

Figure 2.2. Lung volumes. Note that the functional residual capacity and residual volume cannot be measured with the spirometer.

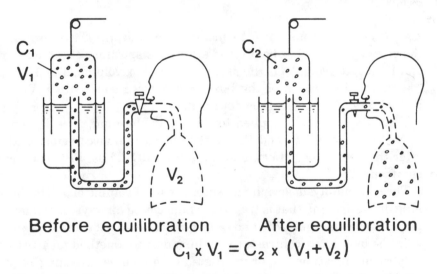

Before equilibration   **After equilibration**

$$C_1 \times V_1 = C_2 \times (V_1 + V_2)$$

Figure 2.3. Measurement of the functional residual capacity by helium dilution.

is with a body plethysmograph (Figure 2.4). This is a large airtight box, like a telephone booth, in which the subject sits. At the end of a normal expiration, a shutter closes the mouthpiece and the subject is asked to make respiratory efforts. As he tries to inhale he expands the gas in his lungs, lung volume increases, and the box pressure rises since its gas volume decreases. Boyle's law states that pres-

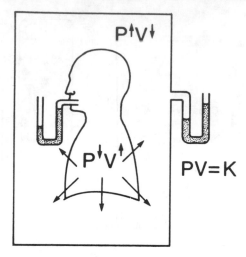

Figure 2.4. Measurement of FRC with a body plethysmograph. When the subject makes an inspiratory effort against a closed airway, he slightly increases the volume of his lung, airway pressure decreases, and box pressure increases. From Boyle's law, lung volume is obtained (see text).

sure × volume is constant (at constant temperature). Therefore, if the pressures in the box before and after the inspiratory effort are P_1 and P_2, respectively, V_1 is the preinspiratory box volume, and ΔV is the change in volume of the box (or lung), we can write $P_1V_1 = P_2(V_1 - \Delta V)$. Thus ΔV can be obtained.

Next, Boyle's law is applied to the gas in the lung. Now $P_3V_2 = P_4(V_2 + \Delta V)$, where P_3 and P_4 are the mouth pressures before and after the inspiratory effort, and V_2 is the FRC. Thus, FRC can be obtained.

The body plethysmograph measures the total volume of gas in the lung, including any that is trapped behind closed airways (for example, as shown in Figure 7.9) and that therefore does not communicate with the mouth. By contrast, the helium dilution method measures only communicating gas, or ventilated lung volume. In young normal subjects these volumes are virtually the same, but in patients with lung disease the ventilated volume may be considerably less than the total volume because of gas trapped behind obstructed airways.

VENTILATION

Suppose the volume exhaled with each breath is 500 ml (Figure 2.1) and there are 15 breaths/min. Then the total volume leaving the lung each minute is $500 \times 15 = 7500$ ml/min. This is known as the total ventilation or minute volume. The volume of air entering the lung is very slightly greater because more oxygen is taken in than carbon dioxide is given out.

However, not all the air that passes the lips reaches the alveolar gas compartment where gas exchange occurs. Of each 500 ml inhaled in Figure 2.1, 150 ml remain behind in the anatomic dead space. Thus, the volume of fresh gas entering the respiratory zone each minute is $(500 - 150) \times 15$ or 5250 ml/min. This is called the *alveolar ventilation* and is of key importance because it represents the amount of fresh inspired air available for gas exchange. (Strictly, the alveolar ventilation is also measured on expiration but the volume is almost the same.)

The total ventilation can easily be measured by having the subject breathe through a valve box that separates the inspired from the expired gas, and collecting all the expired gas in a bag. The alveolar ventilation is more difficult to determine. One way is to measure the volume of the anatomic dead space (see below) and calculate the dead space ventilation (volume × respiratory frequency). This is then subtracted from the total ventilation.

We can summarize this conveniently with symbols (Figure 2.5). Using V to denote volume, and the subscripts T, D, and A to denote tidal, dead space, and alveolar, respectively:

$$V_T = V_D + V_A*$$

therefore
$$V_T \cdot n = V_D \cdot n + V_A \cdot n$$

where n is the respiratory frequency.

Therefore
$$\dot{V}_E = \dot{V}_D + \dot{V}_A$$

where $\dot{V}$ means volume per unit time, $\dot{V}_E$ is expired total ventilation, and $\dot{V}_D$ and $\dot{V}_A$ are the dead space and alveolar ventilations, respectively (see Appendix for a summary of symbols).

Thus
$$\dot{V}_A = \dot{V}_E - \dot{V}_D$$

A difficulty with this method is that the anatomic dead space is not easy to measure, although a value for it can be assumed with little error.

---

*Note that V_A here means the volume of alveolar gas in the tidal volume, not the total volume of alveolar gas in the lung.

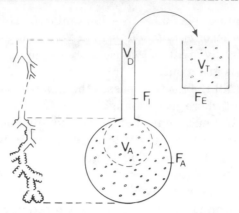

Figure 2.5. The tidal volume (V_T) is a mixture of gas from the anatomic dead space (V_D) and a contribution from the alveolar gas (V_A). The concentrations of CO_2 are shown by the *dots*. F, fractional concentration; I, inspired; E, expired. Compare Figure 1.4. (Modified from J Piiper.)

Another way of measuring alveolar ventilation in normal subjects is from the concentration of CO_2 in expired gas (Figure 2.5). Since no gas exchange occurs in the anatomic dead space, there is no CO_2 there at the end of inspiration. (We can neglect the extremely small amount of CO_2 in the air.) Thus, since all the expired CO_2 comes from the alveolar gas

$$\dot{V}_{CO_2} = \dot{V}_A \times \frac{\% \ CO_2}{100}$$

where $\dot{V}_{CO_2}$ means the volume of CO_2 exhaled per unit time.

Therefore
$$\dot{V}_A = \frac{\dot{V}_{CO_2} \times 100}{\% \ CO_2}$$

The $\% \ CO_2/100$ is often called the fractional concentration and is denoted by F_{CO_2}. Thus the alveolar ventilation can be obtained by dividing the CO_2 output by the alveolar fractional concentration of this gas. The last can be obtained from the final portion of a single expiration by using a rapid CO_2 analyzer.

Note that the partial pressure of CO_2 (denoted P_{CO_2}) is proportional to the fractional concentration of the gas in the alveoli, or $P_{CO_2} = F_{CO_2} \times K$ where K is a constant.

Therefore
$$\dot{V}_A = \frac{\dot{V}_{CO_2}}{P_{CO_2}} \times K$$

$$P_{ACO_2} = \frac{\dot{V}_{CO_2}}{\dot{V}_A} \times K$$

Since in normal subjects the P_{CO_2} of alveolar gas and arterial blood are virtually identical, the arterial P_{CO_2} can be used to determine alveolar ventilation. The relation between alveolar ventilation and P_{CO_2} is of crucial importance. For example, if the alveolar ventilation is halved (and CO_2 production remains unchanged), the alveolar and arterial P_{CO_2} will double.

ANATOMIC DEAD SPACE

This is the volume of the conducting airways (Figures 1.3 and 1.4). The normal value is about 150 ml, and it increases with large inspirations because of the traction exerted on the bronchi by the surrounding lung parenchyma. The dead space also depends on the size and posture of the subject; a rule of thumb is that the volume in milliliters of the seated subject is approximately equal to the body weight in pounds.

The volume of the anatomic dead space can be measured by *Fowler's method*. The subject breathes through a valve box, and the sampling tube of a rapid nitrogen analyzer continuously samples gas at the lips (Figure 2.6A). Following a single inspiration of 100% O_2, the N_2 concentration rises as the dead space gas is increasingly washed out by alveolar gas. Finally, an almost uniform gas concentration is seen representing pure alveolar gas. This phase is often called the alveolar "plateau," although in normal subjects it is not quite flat and in patients with lung diseases it may rise steeply. Expired volume is also recorded.

The dead space is found by plotting N_2 concentration against expired volume and drawing a vertical line such that area A is equal to area B in Figure 2.6B. The dead space is the volume expired up to the vertical line. In effect, this method measures the volume of the conducting airways down to the midpoint of the transition from dead space to alveolar gas.

PHYSIOLOGIC DEAD SPACE

Another way of measuring dead space is *Bohr's method*. Figure 2.5 shows that all the expired CO_2 comes from the alveolar gas and none from the dead space. Therefore we can write

$$V_T \cdot F_E = V_A \cdot F_A$$

now
$$V_T = V_A + V_D$$

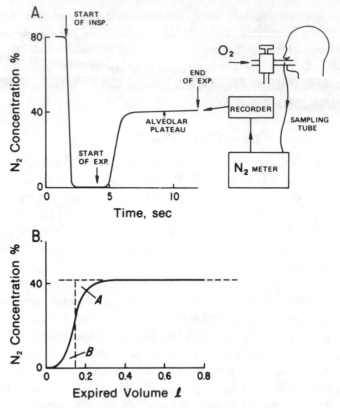

Figure 2.6. Fowler's method of measuring the anatomic dead space with a rapid N_2 analyzer. A shows that following a test inspiration of 100% O_2, the N_2 concentration rises during expiration to an almost level "plateau" representing pure alveolar gas. In B, N_2 concentration is plotted against expired volume, and the dead space is the volume up to the *vertical dashed line* which makes the *areas A and B* equal.

therefore

$$V_A = V_T - V_D$$

substituting

$$V_T \cdot F_E = (V_T - V_D) \cdot F_A$$

whence

$$\frac{V_D}{V_T} = \frac{F_A - F_E}{F_A}$$

We saw earlier that the partial pressure of a gas is proportional to its concentration. Thus

$$\frac{V_D}{V_T} = \frac{P_{A_{CO_2}} - P_{E_{CO_2}}}{P_{A_{CO_2}}} \qquad \text{(Bohr equation)}$$

where A and E refer to alveolar and mixed expired, respectively (see Appendix). The normal ratio of dead space to tidal volume is in the range 0.2–0.35 during resting breathing. In normal subjects, the

P_{CO_2} in alveolar gas and arterial blood are virtually identical so that the equation is therefore often written

$$\frac{V_D}{V_T} = \frac{PA_{CO_2} - PE_{CO_2}}{PA_{CO_2}}$$

It should be noted that Fowler's and Bohr's methods measure somewhat different things. Fowler's method measures the volume of the conducting airways down to the level where the rapid dilution of inspired gas occurs with gas already in the lung. This volume is determined by the geometry of the rapidly expanding airways (Figure 1.5), and because it reflects the morphology of the lung, it is called the *anatomic dead space*. Bohr's method measures the volume of the lung which does not eliminate CO_2. Because this is a functional measurement, the volume is called the *physiologic dead space*. In normal subjects the volumes are very nearly the same. However, in patients with lung disease the physiologic dead space may be considerably larger because of inequality of blood flow and ventilation within the lung (see Chapter 5).

REGIONAL DIFFERENCES IN VENTILATION

So far we have been assuming that all regions of the normal lung have the same ventilation. However, it has been shown that the lower regions of the lung ventilate better than the upper zones. This can be demonstrated if a subject inhales radioactive xenon gas (Figure 2.7). When the xenon-133 enters the counting field, its radiation

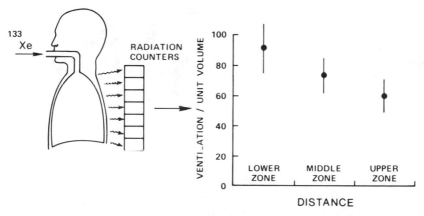

Figure 2.7. Measurement of regional differences in ventilation with radioactive xenon. When the gas is inhaled, its radiation can be detected by counters outside the chest. Note that the ventilation decreases from the lower to upper regions of the upright lung.

penetrates the chest wall and can be recorded by a bank of counters or a radiation camera. In this way the volume of the inhaled xenon going to various regions can be determined.

Figure 2.7 shows the results obtained in a series of normal volunteers using this method. It can be seen that ventilation per unit volume is greatest near the bottom of the lung and becomes progressively smaller toward the top. Other measurements show that when the subject is in the supine position, this difference disappears with the result that apical and basal ventilations become the same. However, in that posture, the ventilation of the lowermost (posterior) lung exceeds that of the uppermost (anterior) lung. Again in the lateral position (subject on his side) the dependent lung is best ventilated. The cause of these regional differences in ventilation will be dealt with in Chapter 7.

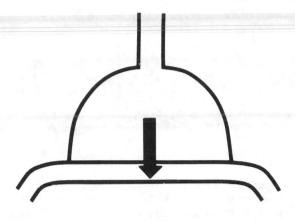

chapter **3**

Diffusion

how gas gets across the alveolar walls

In the last chapter, we looked at how gas is moved from the atmosphere to the alveoli, or in the reverse direction. We now come to the transfer of gas across the blood-gas barrier. This process occurs by *diffusion*. Only 50 years ago, some physiologists believed that the lung secreted oxygen into the capillaries, that is, the oxygen was moved from a region of lower to one of higher partial pressure. Such a process was thought to occur in the swim bladder of fish, and it requires energy. But more accurate measurement showed that this does not occur in the lung and that all gases move across the alveolar wall by passive diffusion.

LAWS OF DIFFUSION

Diffusion through tissues is described by Fick's law (Figure 3.1). This states that the rate of transfer of a gas through a sheet of tissue is proportional to the tissue area and the difference in gas partial

21

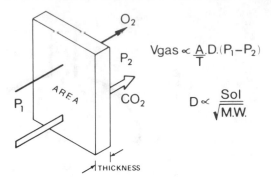

Figure 3.1. Diffusion through a tissue sheet. The amount of gas transferred is proportional to the area (A), a diffusion constant (D), and the difference in partial pressure, and is inversely proportional to the thickness (T). The constant is proportional to the gas solubility (Sol) but inversely proportional to the square root of its molecular weight (MW).

pressure between the two sides, and inversely proportional to the tissue thickness. As we have seen, the area of the blood-gas barrier in the lung is enormous (some 50–100 square meters), and the thickness is less than ½ micron in many places (Figure 1.1), so the dimensions of the barrier are ideal for diffusion. In addition, the rate of transfer is proportional to a diffusion constant which depends on the properties of the tissue and the particular gas. The constant is proportional to the solubility of the gas and inversely proportional to the square root of the molecular weight (Figure 3.1). This means that CO_2 diffuses about 20 times more rapidly than O_2 through tissue sheets since it has a much higher solubility but not a very different molecular weight.

DIFFUSION AND PERFUSION LIMITATIONS

Suppose a red blood cell enters a pulmonary capillary of an alveolus which contains a foreign gas such as carbon monoxide or nitrous oxide. How rapidly will the partial pressure in the blood rise? Figure 3.2 shows the time courses as the red blood cell moves through the capillary, a process that takes about ¾ sec. Look first at carbon monoxide. When the red cell enters the capillary, carbon monoxide moves rapidly across the extremely thin blood-gas barrier from the alveolar gas into the cell. As a result, the content of carbon monoxide in the cell rises. However, because of the tight bond which forms between carbon monoxide and hemoglobin within the cell, a large amount of carbon monoxide can be taken up by the cell with almost

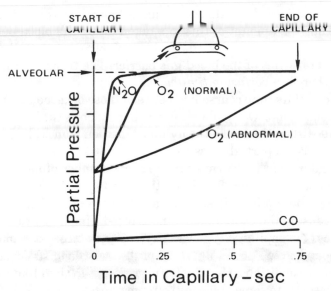

START OF
CAPILLARY

END OF
CAPILLARY

Figure 3.2. Uptake of carbon monoxide, nitrous oxide, and O_2 along the pulmonary capillary. Note that the blood partial pressure of nitrous oxide virtually reaches that of alveolar gas very early in the capillary so that the transfer of this gas is perfusion limited. By contrast, the partial pressure of carbon monoxide in the blood is almost unchanged so that its transfer is diffusion limited. O_2 transfer can be perfusion limited or partly diffusion limited, depending on the conditions.

no increase in partial pressure. Thus, as the cell moves through the capillary, the carbon monoxide partial pressure in the blood hardly changes so that no appreciable back pressure develops, and the gas continues to move rapidly across the alveolar wall. It is clear, therefore, that the amount of carbon monoxide that gets into the blood is limited by the diffusion properties of the blood-gas barrier and not by the amount of blood available.* The transfer of carbon monoxide is therefore said to be *diffusion limited.*

Contrast the time course of nitrous oxide. When this gas moves across the alveolar wall into the blood, no combination with hemoglobin takes place. As a result the blood has nothing like the avidity for nitrous oxide that it has for carbon monoxide, and the partial pressure rises rapidly. Indeed Figure 3.2 shows that the partial pressure of nitrous oxide in the blood has virtually reached that of the alveolar gas by the time the red cell is only one-tenth of the way

---

*This introductory description of carbon monoxide transfer is not completely accurate because of the rate of reaction of carbon monoxide with hemoglobin (see later).

along the capillary. After this point, almost no nitrous oxide is transferred. Thus the amount of this gas taken up by the blood depends entirely on the amount of available blood flow and not at all on the diffusion properties of the blood-gas barrier. The transfer of nitrous oxide is therefore *perfusion limited.*

What of O_2? Its time course lies between those of carbon monoxide and nitrous oxide. O_2 combines with hemoglobin (unlike nitrous oxide) but with nothing like the avidity of carbon monoxide. In other words, the rise in partial pressure when O_2 enters a red blood cell is much greater than is the case for the same number of molecules of carbon monoxide. Figure 3.2 shows that the P_{O_2} of the red blood cell as it enters the capillary is already about four-tenths of the alveolar value because of the O_2 in mixed venous blood. Under typical resting conditions, the capillary P_{O_2} virtually reaches that of alveolar gas when the red cell is about one-third of the way along the capillary. Under these conditions, O_2 transfer is perfusion limited like nitrous oxide. However, in some abnormal circumstances when the diffusion properties of the lung are impaired, for example, because of thickening of the avleolar wall, the blood P_{O_2} does not reach the alveolar value by the end of the capillary, and now there is some diffusion limitation as well.

OXYGEN UPTAKE ALONG THE PULMONARY CAPILLARY

Let us take a closer look at the uptake of O_2 by blood as it moves through a pulmonary capillary. Figure 3.3A shows that the P_{O_2} in a red blood cell entering the capillary is normally about 40 mm Hg. Across the blood-gas barrier, less than ½ micron away, is the alveolar P_{O_2} of 100 mm Hg. Oxygen floods down this large pressure gradient, and the P_{O_2} in the red cell rapidly rises; indeed, as we have seen, it very nearly reaches the P_{O_2} of alveolar gas by the time the red cell is only one-third of its way along the capillary. Thus, under normal circumstances, the difference in P_{O_2} between alveolar gas and end-capillary blood is immeasurably small—a mere fraction of a mm Hg. In other words, the diffusion reserves of the normal lung are enormous.

On severe exercise the pulmonary blood flow is greatly increased, and the time normally spent by the red cell in the capillary, about ¾ sec, may be reduced to as little as one-third of this. Therefore the time available for oxygenation is less, but in normal subjects breathing air there is generally still no measurable fall in end-capillary P_{O_2}.

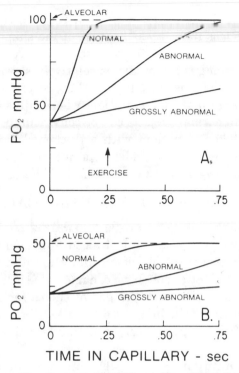

Figure 3.3. Oxygen time courses in the pulmonary capillary when diffusion is normal and abnormal (for example, because of thickening of the alveolar membrane by disease). *A* shows time courses when the alveolar P_{O_2} is normal. *B* shows slower oxygenation when the alveolar P_{O_2} is abnormally low. Note that in both cases, severe exercise reduces the time available for oxygenation.

However, if the blood-gas barrier is markedly thickened by disease so that oxygen diffusion is impeded, the rate of rise of P_{O_2} in the red blood cells is correspondingly slow, and the P_{O_2} may not reach that of alveolar gas before the time available for oxygenation in the capillary has run out. In this case, a measurable difference between alveolar gas and end-capillary blood for P_{O_2} may occur.

Another way of stressing the diffusion properties of the lung is to lower the alveolar P_{O_2} (Figure 3.3*B*). Suppose that this has been reduced to 50 mm Hg, either by the subject going to high altitude, or by giving him a low O_2 mixture to breathe. Now although the P_{O_2} in the red cell at the start of the capillary may only be about 20 mm Hg, the partial pressure difference responsible for driving the O_2 across the blood-gas barrier has been reduced from 60 mm Hg (Figure 3.3*A*) to only 30 mm Hg. O_2 therefore moves across more slowly. In addition, the rate of rise of P_{O_2} for a given increase in O_2 concentration in the blood is less than it was because of the shape of the O_2 dissociation curve (see Chapter 6). For both of these reasons, therefore, the rise in P_{O_2} along the capillary is relatively slow, and failure to reach the alveolar P_{O_2} is more likely. Thus, severe exercise at very high altitude is one of the few situations where diffusion impairment of O_2 transfer in normal subjects can be convincingly demonstrated. By the same token, a patient with a thickened blood-gas barrier will be most likely to show evidence of diffusion impairment if he breathes a low oxygen mixture, especially if he exercises as well.

MEASUREMENT OF DIFFUSING CAPACITY

We have seen that oxygen transfer into the pulmonary capillary is normally limited by the amount of blood flow available, although under some circumstances diffusion limitation also occurs (Figure 3.2). By contrast, the transfer of carbon monoxide is limited solely by diffusion, and it is therefore the gas of choice for measuring the diffusion properties of the lung. At one time O_2 was employed under hypoxic conditions (Figure 3.3B), but this technique is no longer used.

The laws of diffusion (Figure 3.1) state that the amount of gas transferred across a sheet of tissue is proportional to the area, a diffusion constant, and the difference in partial pressure, and inversely proportional to the thickness, or

$$\dot{V}gas = \frac{A}{T} \cdot D \cdot (P_1 - P_2)$$

Now for a complex structure like the blood-gas barrier of the lung, it is not possible to measure the area and thickness during life. Instead, the equation is rewritten

$$\dot{V}gas = D_L \cdot (P_1 - P_2)$$

where D_L is called the *diffusing capacity of the lung* and includes the area, thickness, and diffusion properties of the sheet and the gas concerned. Thus the diffusing capacity for carbon monoxide is given by

$$D_L = \frac{\dot{V}_{CO}}{P_1 - P_2}$$

where P_1 and P_2 are the partial pressures of alveolar gas and capillary blood, respectively. But as we have seen (Figure 3.2), the partial pressure of carbon monoxide in capillary blood is extremely small and it can generally be neglected. Thus

$$D_L = \frac{\dot{V}_{CO}}{P_{A_{CO}}}$$

or, in words, the diffusing capacity of the lung for carbon monoxide is the volume of carbon monoxide transferred in milliliters per minute per mm Hg of alveolar partial pressure.

Several techniques for making this measurement are available. In the *single breath method,* a single inspiration of a dilute mixture of carbon monoxide is made, and the rate of disappearance of carbon monoxide from the alveolar gas during a 10-sec breathhold is calculated. This is usually done by measuring the inspired and expired concentrations of carbon monoxide with an infrared analyzer. The alveolar concentration of carbon monoxide is not constant during the breathholding period, but allowance can be made for that. Helium is also added to the inspired gas to give a measurement of lung volume by dilution.

In the *steady state method,* the subject breathes a low concentration of carbon monoxide (about 0.1%) for ½ min or so until a steady state has been reached. The constant rate of disappearance of carbon monoxide from alveolar gas is then measured for a further short period along with the alveolar concentration. The normal value of the diffusing capacity for carbon monoxide at rest is about 25 ml/min/mm Hg, and it increases to two or three times this value on exercise.

REACTION RATES WITH HEMOGLOBIN

So far we have assumed that all the resistance to the movement of O_2 and CO resides in the barrier between blood and gas. However, Figure 1.1 shows that the path length from the alveolar wall to the center of a red blood cell exceeds that in the wall itself so that some of the diffusion resistance is located within the capillary. In addition, there is another type of resistance to gas transfer that is most conveniently discussed with diffusion, that is, the resistance caused by the finite rate of reaction of O_2 or CO with hemoglobin inside the red blood cell.

When O_2 (or CO) is added to blood, its combination with hemoglobin is quite fast, being well on the way to completion in ⅕ sec. However, oxygenation occurs so rapidly in the pulmonary capillary (Figure 3.3) that even this rapid reaction significantly delays the loading of O_2 by the red cell. Thus, the uptake of O_2 (or CO) can be regarded as occurring in two stages: (1) diffusion of O_2 through the blood-gas barrier (including the plasma and red cell interior); and (2) reaction of the O_2 with hemoglobin (Figure 3.4). In fact it is possible to sum the two resultant resistances to produce an overall "diffusion" resistance.

We saw that the diffusing capacity of the lung is defined as $D_L = \dot{V}gas/(P_1 - P_2)$, that is, as the flow of gas divided by a pressure difference. Thus the inverse of D_L is pressure difference divided by flow and is therefore analogous to electrical resistance. Consequently, the resistance of the blood-gas barrier in Figure 3.4 is shown as $1/D_M$, where M means membrane. Now the rate of reaction of O_2 (or CO) with hemoglobin can be described by θ, which gives the rate in ml per minute of O_2 (or CO) which combine with 1 ml of blood per mm Hg partial pressure of O_2 (or CO). This is analogous to the "diffusing capacity" of 1 ml of blood and, when multiplied by the volume of capillary blood (V_C), gives the effective "diffusing capacity" of the rate of reaction of O_2 with hemoglobin. Again its inverse, $1/(\theta \cdot V_C)$ describes the resistance of this reaction. We can add the resistances offered by the membrane and the blood to obtain the total diffusion resistance. Thus the complete equation is

$$\frac{1}{D_L} = \frac{1}{D_M} + \frac{1}{\theta \cdot V_C}$$

In practice, the resistances offered by the membrane and blood components are approximately equal so that a reduction of capillary

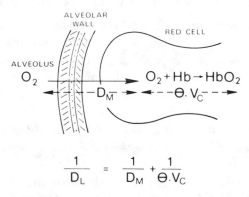

$$\frac{1}{D_L} = \frac{1}{D_M} + \frac{1}{\theta \cdot V_C}$$

Figure 3.4. The diffusing capacity of the lung (D_L) is made up of two components, that due to the diffusion process itself and that attributable to the time taken for O_2 (or CO) to react with hemoglobin.

blood volume by disease can reduce the diffusing capacity of the lung

INTERPRETATION OF DIFFUSING CAPACITY FOR CO

It is clear that the measured diffusing capacity of the lung for CO depends not only on the area and thickness of the blood-gas barrier but also on the volume of blood in the pulmonary capillaries. Futhermore, in the diseased lung, the measurement is affected by the distribution of diffusion properties, alveolar volume, and capillary blood. For these reasons, the term transfer factor is sometimes used (particularly in Europe) to emphasize that the measurement does not solely reflect the diffusion properties of the lung.

CO_2 TRANSFER ACROSS THE PULMONARY CAPILLARY

We have seen that of diffusion of CO_2 through tissue is about 20 times faster than that of O_2 because of the much higher solubility of CO_2 (Figure 3.1). At first sight, therefore, it seems unlikely that CO_2 elimination could be affected by diffusion difficulties, and indeed this has been the general belief. However, the reaction of CO_2 with

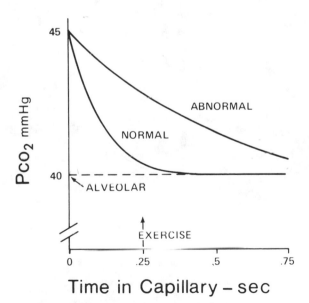

Time in Capillary – sec

Figure 3.5. Calculated changes in P_{CO_2} along the capillary when the diffusion properties are normal and abnormal (compare the time course of P_{O_2} in Figure 3.3). (From PD Wagner and JB West: *J Appl Physiol* 33:62, 1972.)

blood is complex (see Chapter 6), and although there is some uncertainty about the rates of the various reactions, it is possible that a difference between end-capillary blood and alveolar gas can develop if the blood-gas barrier is diseased.

Figure 3.5 shows the normal time course for CO_2 and how it might be affected by thickening of the blood-gas barrier. Note that the P_{CO_2} of the blood as it enters the capillary is about 45 mm Hg and that the normal P_{CO_2} of alveolar gas is about 40 mm Hg. It can be seen that the time taken for the blood to reach virtually the same partial pressure as alveolar gas is similar to that for O_2 under normal conditions (Figure 3.3), so that there are good reserves of diffusion. However, when the diffusing capacity of the membrane is reduced to about one-fourth of its normal value, a small difference between end-capillary blood and alveolar gas may be seen.

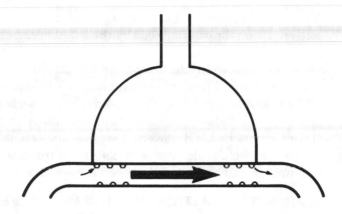

chapter 4

Blood Flow and Metabolism

*how the blood vessels remove gas
from the lung and alter some
compounds*

The pulmonary circulation begins at the main pulmonary artery, which receives the mixed venous blood pumped by the right ventricle. This artery then branches successively like the system of airways (Figure 1.3), and indeed the pulmonary arteries accompany the bronchi down the center of the secondary lobules as far as the terminal bronchioles. Beyond that they break up to supply the capillary bed, which lies in the walls of the alveoli (Figures 1.6 and 1.7). The pulmonary capillaries form a dense network in the alveolar wall which makes an exceedingly efficient arrangement for gas exchange (Figures 1.1, 1.6, and 1.7). So rich is the mesh that some physiologists feel that it is misleading to talk of a network of individual capillary segments and prefer to regard the capillary bed as a sheet of flowing blood interrupted in places by posts (Figure 1.6), rather like an underground parking garage. The oxygenated blood is then collected from the capillary bed by the small pulmonary veins which run between the lobules and eventually unite to form the four large veins (in man) which drain into the left atrium.

At first sight, this circulation appears to be simply a small version of the systemic circulation which begins at the aorta and ends in the right atrium. Indeed, the pulmonary circulation is often called the "lesser circulation." However, there are important differences between the two circulations, and confusion frequently results from attempts to emphasize similarities between them.

PRESSURES WITHIN PULMONARY BLOOD VESSELS

The pressures in the pulmonary circulation are remarkably low. The mean pressure in the main pulmonary artery is only about 15 mm Hg; the systolic and diastolic pressures are about 25 and 8 mm Hg, respectively (Figure 4.1). The pressure is therefore very pulsatile. By contrast the mean pressure in the aorta is about 100 mm Hg—about six times more than in the pulmonary artery. The pressures in the right and left atriums are not very dissimilar—about 2 and 5 mm Hg, respectively. Thus the pressure differences from inlet to outlet of the pulmonary and systemic systems are about $(15 - 5) = 10$ and $(100 - 2) = 98$ mm Hg, respectively—a factor of 10.

In keeping with these low pressures, the walls of the pulmonary artery and its branches are remarkably thin and contain relatively

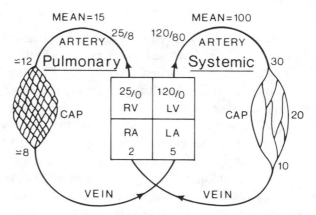

Figure 4.1. Comparison of pressures (mm Hg) in the pulmonary and systemic circulations. Hydrostatic differences modify these.

little smooth muscle (they are easily mistaken for veins). This is in striking contrast to the systemic circulation where the arteries generally have thick walls, and the arterioles in particular have abundant smooth muscle.

The reasons for these differences become clear when the functions of the two circulations are compared. The systemic circulation regulates the supply of blood to various organs, including those which may be far above the level of the heart (the upstretched arm, for example). By contrast, the lung is required to accept the whole of the cardiac output at all times. It is rarely concerned with directing blood from one region to another (an exception is localized alveolar hypoxia, see below), and its arterial pressure is therefore as low as is consistent with lifting blood to the top of the lung. This keeps the work of the right heart as small as is feasible for efficient gas exchange to occur in the lung.

The pressure within the pulmonary capillaries is uncertain. Several pieces of evidence suggest that it lies about halfway between pulmonary arterial and venous pressure, and some work indicates that much of the pressure drop occurs within the capillary bed itself. Certainly the distribution of pressures along the pulmonary circulation is far more symmetrical than in its systemic counterpart, where most of the pressure drop is just upstream of the capillaries (Figure 4.1). In addition, the pressure within the pulmonary capillaries varies considerably throughout the lung because of hydrostatic effects (see below).

PRESSURES AROUND PULMONARY BLOOD VESSELS

The pulmonary capillaries are unique in that they are virtually surrounded by gas (Figures 1.1 and 1.7). It is true that there is a very thin layer of epithelial cells lining the alveoli, but the capillaries receive little support from this and, consequently, they are liable to collapse or distend, depending on the pressures within and around them. The latter is very close to alveolar pressure. (The pressure in the alveoli is usually close to atmospheric pressure; indeed, during breathholding with the glottis open, the two pressures are identical.) Under some special conditions, the effective pressure around the capillaries is reduced by the surface tension of the fluid lining the alveoli. But usually, the effective pressure is alveolar pressure, and when this rises above the pressure inside the capillaries, they collapse. The pressure difference between the inside and outside of the vessels is often called the *transmural pressure*.

What is the pressure around the pulmonary arteries and veins? This can be considerably less than alveolar pressure. As the lung expands, these larger blood vessels are pulled open by the radial traction of the elastic lung parenchyma which surrounds them (Figures 4.2 and 4.3). Consequently, the effective pressure around them is low; in fact there is some evidence that this pressure is even less than the pressure around the whole lung (intrapleural pressure). This paradox can be explained by the mechanical advantage that

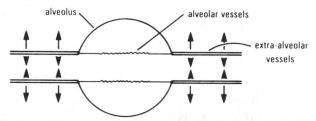

Figure 4.2. "Alveolar" and "extra-alveolar" vessels. The first are mainly the capillaries and are exposed to alveolar pressure. The second are pulled open by the radial traction of the surrounding lung parenchyma, and the effective pressure around them is therefore lower than alveolar pressure. (From JMB Hughes et al: *Respir Physiol* 4:58, 1968.)

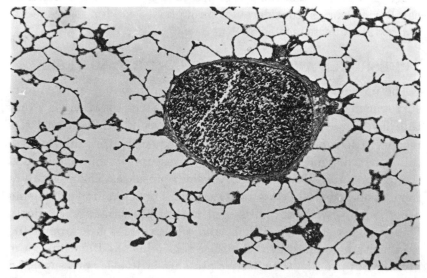

Figure 4.3. Section of lung showing many alveoli and an extra-alveolar vessel (in this case, a small vein) with its perivascular sheath.

develops when a relatively rigid structure like a blood vessel or bronchus is surrounded by a rapidly expanding elastic material such as lung parenchyma. In any event, both the arteries and veins increase their caliber as the lung expands.

The behavior of the capillaries and the larger blood vessels is so different they they are often referred to as alveolar and extra-alveolar vessels (Figure 4.2). Alveolar vessels are exposed to alveolar pressure and include the capillaries and the slightly larger vessels in the corners of the alveolar walls. Their caliber is determined by the relationship between alveolar pressure and the pressure within them. Extra-alveolar vessels include all the arteries and veins which run through the lung parenchyma. Their caliber is greatly affected by lung volume since this determines the expanding pull of the parenchyma on their walls. The very large vessels near the hilum are outside the lung substance and are exposed to intrapleural pressure.

PULMONARY VASCULAR RESISTANCE

It is useful to describe the resistance of a system of blood vessels as follows:

$$\text{Vascular resistance} = \frac{\text{input pressure} - \text{output pressure}}{\text{blood flow}}$$

This number is certainly not a complete description of the pressure-flow properties of the system. For example, the number usually depends on the magnitude of the blood flow. Nevertheless, it often allows a helpful comparison of different circulations, or the same circulation under different conditions.

We have seen that the total pressure drop from pulmonary artery to left atrium in the pulmonary circulation is only some 10 mm Hg against about 100 mm Hg for the systemic circulation. Since the blood flows through the two circulations are virtually identical, it follows that the pulmonary vascular resistance is only one-tenth that of the systemic circulation. The pulmonary blood flow is about 6 liters/min so that, in numbers, the pulmonary vascular resistance = (15 − 5)/6 or about 1.7 mm Hg/liter/min.* The high resistance of the systemic circulation is is largely caused by the muscular arterioles which allow the regulation of blood flow to various

---

*Cardiologists sometimes express pulmonary vascular resistance in the units dynes · sec · cm^{-5}. The normal value is then in the region of 100.

organs of the body. The pulmonary circulation has no such vessels and appears to have as low a resistance as is compatible with distributing the blood in a thin film over a vast area in the alveolar walls.

Although the normal pulmonary vascular resistance is extraordinarily small, it has a remarkable facility for becoming even smaller as the pressure within it rises. Figure 4.4 shows that an increase in either pulmonary arterial or venous pressure causes pulmonary vascular resistance to fall. Two mechanisms are responsible for this. Under normal conditions, some capillaries are either closed, or open but with no blood flow. As the pressure rises, these vessels begin to conduct blood, thus lowering the overall resistance. This is termed *recruitment* (Figure 4.5) and is apparently the chief mechanism for the fall in pulmonary vascular resistance that occurs as the pulmonary artery pressure is raised from low levels. The reason why some vessels are unperfused at low perfusing pressures is not fully understood but perhaps is caused by random differences in the geometry of the complex network (Figure 1.3) which result in preferential channels for flow.

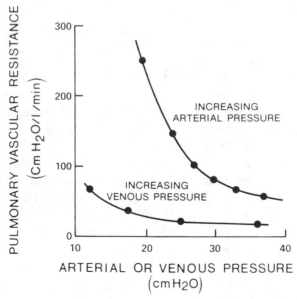

Figure 4.4. Fall in pulmonary vascular resistance as the pulmonary arterial or venous pressure is raised. When the arterial pressure was changed, the venous pressure was held constant at 12 cm water, and when the venous pressure was changed, the arterial pressure was held at 37 cm water. (Data from an excised dog lung preparation.)

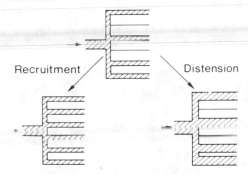

Figure 4.5. Recruitment (opening up of previously closed vessels) and distension (increase in caliber of vessels). These are the two mechanisms for the decrease in pulmonary vascular resistance that occurs as vascular pressures are raised.

At higher vascular pressures, widening of individual capillary segments occurs. This increase in caliber, or *distension*, is hardly surprising in view of the very thin membrane which separates the capillary from the alveolar space (Figure 1.1). Distension is apparently the predominant mechanism for the fall in pulmonary vascular resistance at relatively high vascular pressures.

Another important determinant of pulmonary vascular resistance is *lung volume*. The caliber of the extra-alveolar vessels (Figure 4.2) is determined by a balance between various forces. As we have seen, they are pulled open as the lung expands. As a result their vascular resistance is low at large lung volumes. On the other hand, their walls contain smooth muscle and elastic tissue which resist distension and tend to reduce their caliber. Consequently they have a high resistance when lung volume is low (Figure 4.6). Indeed, if the lung is completely collapsed, the smooth muscle tone of these vessels is so effective that the pulmonary artery pressure has to be raised several centimeters of water above downstream pressure before any flow at all occurs. This is called a *critical opening pressure.*

Is the vascular resistance of the capillaries influenced by lung volume? This depends on whether alveolar pressure changes with respect to the pressure inside the capillaries, that is, whether their transmural pressure alters. If alveolar pressure rises with respect to capillary pressure, the vessels tend to be squashed, and their resistance rises. This usually occurs when a normal subject takes a deep inspiration, because the vascular pressures fall. (The heart is surrounded by intrapleural pressure, which falls on inspiration.) However, the pressures in the pulmonary circulation do not remain

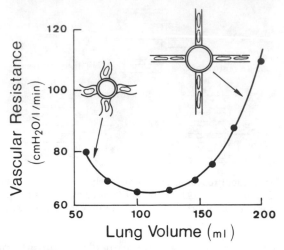

Figure 4.6.   Effect of lung volume on pulmonary vascular resistance when the transmural pressure of the capillaries is held constant. At low lung volumes, resistance is high because the extra-alveolar vessels become narrow. At high volumes, the capillaries are stretched, and their caliber is reduced. (Data from a dog lobe preparation.)

steady after such a maneuver. An additional factor is that the caliber of the capillaries is reduced at large lung volumes because of stretching of the alveolar walls. Thus even if the transmural pressure of the capillaries is not changed with large lung inflations their vascular resistance increases (Figure 4.6).

Because of the role of smooth muscle in determining the caliber of the extra-alveolar vessels, drugs that cause contraction of the muscle increase pulmonary vascular resistance. These include serotonin, histamine, and norepinephrine. These drugs are particularly effective vasoconstrictors when the lung volume is low and the expanding forces on the vessels are weak. Drugs that can relax smooth muscle in the pulmonary circulation include acetylcholine and isoproterenol.

MEASUREMENT OF PULMONARY BLOOD FLOW

The volume of blood passing through the lungs each minute ($\dot{Q}$) can be calculated using the *Fick principle*. This states that the O_2 consumption per minute ($\dot{V}_{O_2}$) is equal to the amount of O_2 taken up by the blood in the lungs per minute. Since the O_2 concentration in the blood entering the lungs is $C\bar{v}_{O_2}$ and that in the blood leaving is Ca_{O_2} we have

$$\dot{V}_{O_2} = \dot{Q}(Ca_{O_2} - C\bar{v}_{O_2})$$

or

$$\dot{Q} = \frac{\dot{V}_{O_2}}{Ca_{O_2} - C\bar{v}_{O_2}}$$

$\dot{V}_{O_2}$ is measured by collecting the expired gas in a large spirometer and measuring its O_2 concentration. Mixed venous blood is taken via a catheter in the pulmonary artery and arterial blood by puncture of the brachial or radial artery. Pulmonary blood flow can also be measured by the indicator dilution technique in which dye, for example, is injected into the venous circulation and its concentration in arterial blood is recorded. Both these methods are of great importance but they will not be considered in more detail here because they fall within the province of cardiovascular physiology.

The Fick and indicator dilution methods give the average flow over a number of heart cycles. It is also possible to measure *instantaneous pulmonary blood flow* using the body plethysmograph (Figure 4.7). For this application the subject inhales a gas mixture containing 79% nitrous oxide and 21% O_2 from a rubber bag inside the box. Nitrous oxide is a very soluble gas, and as it is taken up by the blood, the box pressure falls in a series of small steps which are synchronous with the heartbeat. Since the uptake of nitrous oxide is

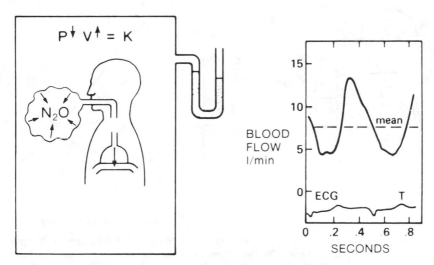

Figure 4.7. Measurement of instantaneous capillary blood flow by recording nitrous oxide uptake in a body plethysmograph. Calculated blood flow is shown on the right with the electrocardiogram.

flow limited (Figure 3.2), instantaneous blood flow can be calculated. In normal subjects, there is considerable pulsatility of pulmonary capillary blood flow; this is altered by disease.

DISTRIBUTION OF BLOOD FLOW

So far we have been assuming that all parts of the pulmonary circulation behave identically. However, considerable inequality of blood flow exists within the human lung. This can be shown by a modification of the radioactive xenon method that was used to measure the distribution of ventilation (Figure 2.7). For the measurement of blood flow, the xenon is dissolved in saline and injected into a peripheral vein (Figure 4.8). When it reaches the pulmonary capillaries it is evolved into alveolar gas because of its low solubility, and the distribution of radioactivity can be measured by counters over the chest during breathholding.

In the upright human lung, blood flow decreases almost linearly from bottom to top, reaching very low values at the apex (Figure 4.8). This distribution is affected by change of posture and exercise. When the subject lies supine, the apical zone blood flow increases but the basal zone flow remains virtually unchanged, with the result that

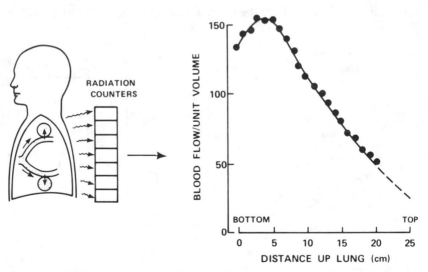

Figure 4.8. Measurement of the distribution of blood flow in the upright human lung using radioactive xenon. The dissolved xenon is evolved into alveolar gas from the pulmonary capillaries. The units of blood flow are such that if flow were uniform, all values would be 100. Note the small flow at the apex. (Redrawn from JMB Hughes et al: *Respir Physiol* 4:58, 1968.)

the distribution from apex to base becomes almost uniform. However, in this posture, blood flow in the posterior (dependent) regions of the lung exceeds flow in the anterior parts. Measurements on men suspended upside down show that apical blood flow may exceed basal flow in this position. On mild exercise, both upper and lower zone blood flows increase, and the regional differences become less.

The uneven distribution of blood flow can be explained by the hydrostatic pressure differences within the blood vessels. If we consider the pulmonary arterial system as a continuous column of blood, the difference in pressure between the top and bottom of a lung 30 cm high will be about 30 cm water, or 23 mm Hg. This is a large pressure difference for such a low pressure system as the pulmonary circulation (Figure 4.1), and its effects on regional blood flow are shown in Figure 4.9.

There may be a region at the top of the lung (*zone 1*) where pulmonary arterial pressure falls below alveolar pressure (normally close to atmospheric pressure). If this occurs, the capillaries are squashed flat, and no flow is possible. This zone 1 does *not* occur under normal conditions because the pulmonary arterial pressure is just sufficient to raise blood to the top of the lung but may be present if the arterial pressure is reduced (following severe hemorrhage, for example) or if alveolar pressure is raised (during positive pressure

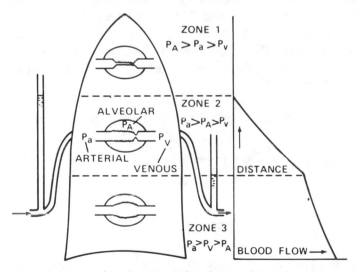

Figure 4.9. Model to explain the uneven distribution of blood flow in the lung based on the pressures affecting the capillaries. (From JB West et al: *J Appl Physiol* 19:713, 1964.)

ventilation). This ventilated but unperfused lung is useless for gas exchange and is called *alveolar dead space*.

Farther down the lung (*zone 2*), pulmonary arterial pressure increases because of the hydrostatic effect and now exceeds alveolar pressure. However, venous pressure is still very low and is less than alveolar pressure, and this leads to remarkable pressure-flow characteristics. Under these conditions blood flow is determined by the difference between arterial and alveolar pressures (not the usual arterial-venous pressure difference). Indeed, venous pressure has no influence on flow unless it exceeds alveolar pressure.

This behavior can be modeled with a flexible rubber tube inside a glass chamber (Figure 4.10). When chamber pressure is greater than downstream pressure, the rubber tube collapses at its downstream end, and the pressure in the tube at this point limits flow. The pulmonary capillary bed is clearly very different from a rubber tube but nevertheless the overall behavior is similar and is often called the Starling resistor, sluice, or waterfall effect. Since arterial pressure is increasing down the zone but alveolar pressure is the same throughout the lung, the pressure difference responsible for flow increases. In addition, increasing recruitment of capillaries occurs down this zone.

In *zone 3*, venous pressure now exceeds alveolar pressure, and flow is determined in the usual way by the arterial-venous pressure difference. The increase in blood flow down this region of the lung is apparently caused chiefly by distension of the capillaries. The pressure within them (lying between arterial and venous) increases down the zone while the pressure outside (alveolar) remains con-

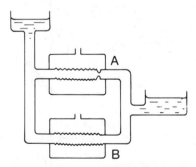

Figure 4.10. Two Starling resistors, each consisting of a thin rubber tube inside a container. When chamber pressure exceeds downstream pressure as in *A*, flow is independent of downstream pressure. However, when downstream pressure exceeds chamber pressure as in *B*, flow is determined by the upstream-downstream difference.

stant. Thus their transmural pressure rises and, indeed, measurements show that their mean width increases. Recruitment of previously closed vessels may also play some part in the increase in blood flow down this zone.

The scheme shown in Figure 4.9 summarizes the role played by the capillaries in determining the distribution of blood flow. At low lung volumes, the resistance of the extra-alveolar vessels becomes important, and a reduction of regional blood flow is seen, starting first at the base of the lung, where the parenchyma is least expanded (see Figure 7.8). This region of reduced blood flow is sometimes called *zone 4* and can be explained by the narrowing of the extra-alveolar vessels which occurs when the lung around them is poorly inflated (Figure 4.6).

HYPOXIC VASOCONSTRICTION

We have seen that passive factors dominate the vascular resistance and the distribution of flow in the pulmonary circulation under normal conditions. However, a remarkable active response occurs when the P_{O_2} of alveolar gas is reduced. This consists of contraction of smooth muscle in the walls of the small arterioles in the hypoxic region. The precise mechanism of this response is obscure, but it occurs in excised isolated lung and so does not depend on central nervous connections. Excised segments of pulmonary artery can be shown to constrict if their environment is made hypoxic so that it may be a local action of the hypoxia on the artery itself. One hypothesis is that cells in the perivascular tissue release some vasoconstrictor substance in response to hypoxia, but an intensive search for the mediator has not been successful. Interestingly, it is the P_{O_2} of the alveolar gas, not the pulmonary arterial blood, that chiefly determines the response. This can be proved by perfusing a lung with blood of a high P_{O_2} while keeping the alveolar P_{O_2} low. Under these conditions the response occurs.

The vessel wall presumably becomes hypoxic through diffusion of oxygen over the very short distance from the wall to the surrounding alveoli. Recall that a small pulmonary artery is very closely surrounded by alveoli (compare the proximity of alveoli to the small pulmonary vein in Figure 4.3). The stimulus-response curve of this constriction is very nonlinear (Figure 4.11). When the alveolar P_{O_2} is altered in the region above 100 mm Hg, little change in vascular resistance is seen. However, when the alveolar P_{O_2} is reduced below

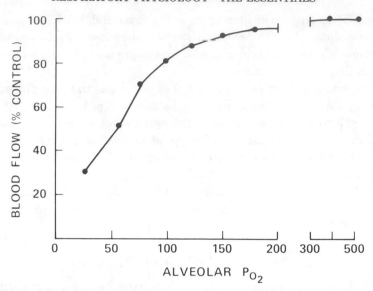

Figure 4.11. Effect of reducing alveolar PO_2 on pulmonary blood flow. Data from anesthetized cat. (From GR Barer et al: *J Physiol* 211:139, 1970.)

approximately 70 mm Hg, marked vasoconstriction may occur, and at a very low P_{O_2} the local blood flow may be almost abolished.

The vasoconstriction has the effect of directing blood flow away from hypoxic regions of lung. These regions may result from bronchial obstruction, and by diverting blood flow the deleterious effects on gas exchange are reduced. At high altitude, generalized pulmonary vasoconstriction may occur, leading to a large rise in pulmonary arterial pressure and a substantial increase in work for the right heart. But probably the most important situation where this mechanism operates is at birth. During fetal life, the pulmonary vascular resistance is very high, partly because of hypoxic vasoconstriction, and only some 15% of the cardiac output goes through the lungs (see Figure 9.5). When the first breath oxygenates the alveoli, the vascular resistance falls dramatically because of relaxation of vascular smooth muscle, and the pulmonary blood flow enormously increases.

Other active responses of the pulmonary circulation have been described. A low blood pH causes vasoconstriction, especially when alveolar hypoxia is present. There is also evidence that the autonomic nervous system exerts a weak control, an increase in sympathetic outflow causing stiffening of the walls of the pulmonary arteries and vasoconstriction.

WATER BALANCE IN THE LUNG

Since only ½ micron of tissue separates the capillary blood from the air in the lung (Figure 1.1), the problem of keeping the alveoli free of fluid is critical. Fluid exchange across the capillary wall is believed to obey Starling's law. The force tending to push fluid *out* of the capillary is the capillary hydrostatic pressure minus the hydrostatic pressure in the interstitital fluid, or $P_c - P_i$. The force tending to pull fluid *in* is the colloid osmotic pressure of the proteins of the blood minus that of the proteins of the interstitial fluid, or $\pi_c - \pi_i$. This force depends on the reflection coefficient σ which indicates the effectiveness of the capillary wall in preventing the passage of proteins across it. Thus

$$\text{net fluid out} = K[(P_c - P_i) - \sigma(\pi_c - \pi_i)]$$

where K is a constant called the filtration coefficient.

Unfortunately, the practical use of this equation is limited because of our ignorance of many of the values. The colloid osmotic pressure within the capillary is about 28 mm Hg. The capillary hydrostatic pressure is probably about halfway between arterial and venous pressure but is much higher at the bottom of the lung than the top. The colloid osmotic pressure of the interstitial fluid is not known but is about 20 mm Hg in lung lymph. However, this value may be higher than that in the interstitital fluid around the capillaries. The interstitial hydrostatic pressure is unknown but is thought by some physiologists to be substantially below atmospheric pressure. It is probable that the net pressure of the Starling equation is outward, causing a small lymph flow of perhaps 20 ml/hr in man under normal conditions.

Where does fluid go when it leaves the capillaries? Figure 4.12 shows that fluid which leaks out into the interstitium of the alveolar wall tracks through the interstitial space to the perivascular and peribronchial space within the lung. Numerous lymphatics run in the perivascular spaces, and these help to transport the fluid to the hilar lymph nodes. In addition, the pressure in these perivascular spaces is low, thus forming a natural sump for the drainage of fluid (compare Figure 4.2). The earliest form of pulmonary edema[†] is char-

---

[†] For a more extended discussion of pulmonary edema, see the companion volume, JB West: *Pulmonary Pathophysiology—the essentials,* ed 3. Baltimore, Williams & Wilkins, 1987.

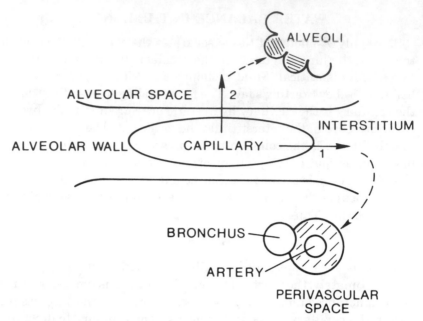

Figure 4.12. Two routes for loss of fluid from pulmonary capillaries. Fluid which enters the interstitium initially finds its way into the perivascular and peribronchial spaces. Later fluid may cross the alveolar wall, filling alveolar spaces.

acterized by engorgement of these peribronchial and perivascular spaces and is known as interstitital edema.

In a later stage of pulmonary edema, fluid crosses the alveolar epithelium into the alveolar spaces (Figure 4.12). When this occurs, the alveoli fill with fluid one by one and, since they are then unventilated, no oxygenation of the blood passing through them is possible. What causes fluid to start moving across into the alveolar spaces is not know, but it may be that this occurs when the maximal drainage rate through the interstitital space is exceeded and the pressure there rises too high. The normal rate of lymph flow from the lung is only a few milliliters per hour but it can be shown to increase greatly if the capillary pressure is raised over a long period. Alveolar edema is much more serious than interstitial edema because of the interference with pulmonary gas exchange.

OTHER FUNCTIONS OF THE PULMONARY CIRCULATION

The chief function of the pulmonary circulation is to move blood to and from the blood-gas barrier so that gas exchange can occur. However, it has other important functions too. One is to act as a reservoir for blood. We saw that the lung has a remarkable ability for reducing its pulmonary vascular resistance as its vascular pressures are raised though the mechanisms of recruitment and distension (Figure 4.5). The same mechanisms allow the lung to increase its blood volume with relatively small rises in pulmonary arterial or venous pressures. This occurs, for example, when a subject lies down after standing. Blood then drains from the legs into the lung.

Another function of the lung is to filter blood. Small blood thrombi are removed from the circulation before they can reach the brain or other vital organs. There is also evidence that many white blood cells are trapped by the lung, although the value of this is not clear.

METABOLIC FUNCTIONS OF THE LUNG

The lung has important metabolic functions in addition to gas exchange. One of the most important of these is the synthesis of phospholipids such as dipalmitoyl phosphatidyl choline, which is a component of pulmonary surfactant (see Chapter 7). Protein synthesis is also clearly important since collagen and elastin form the structural framework of the lung. Under abnormal conditions, proteases are apparently liberated from leukocytes or macrophages in the lung, causing breakdown of proteins and thus emphysema. Another significant area is carbohydrate metabolism, especially the elaboration of mucopolysaccharides of bronchial mucus.

A number of vasoactive substances are metabolized by the lung, as shown in Figure 4.13. Since the lung is the only organ except the heart which receives the whole circulation, it is uniquely suited to modifying blood-borne substances. A substantial fraction of all the vascular endothelial cells in the body are located in the lung.

The only known example of biological activation by passage through the pulmonary circulation is the conversion of the relatively inactive polypeptide, angiotensin I, to the potent vasoconstrictor, angiotensin II. The latter, which is up to 50 times more active than its precursor, is unaffected by passage through the lung. The conversion of angiotensin I is catalyzed by an enzyme, angiotensin-converting enzyme or ACE, which is located in small pits (caveolae intracellulares) in the surface of the capillary endothelial cells.

Many vasoactive substances are completely or partially inactivated during passage through the lung. Bradykinin is largely inactivated (up to 80%), and the enzyme responsible is angiotensin-converting enzyme, ACE. The lung is the major site of inactivation of serotonin (5-hydroxytryptamine), but this is not by enzymatic

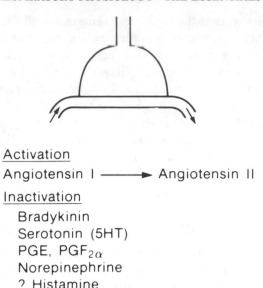

Activation

Angiotensin I ⟶ Angiotensin II

Inactivation

  Bradykinin

  Serotonin (5HT)

  PGE, $PGF_{2\alpha}$

  Norepinephrine

  ? Histamine

Figure 4.13. Pulmonary metabolism of vasoactive substances. The inactivation of bradykinin, serotonin, PGE, and $PGF_{2\alpha}$ is highly effective but only partial for norepinephrine and histamine.

degradation, but by an uptake and storage process. Some of the serotonin may be transferred to platelets in the lung, or stored in some other way and released during anaphylaxis. The prostaglandins E_1, E_2, and $F_{2\alpha}$ are also inactivated in the lung, which is a rich source of the responsible enzymes. Norepinephrine is also taken up by the lung to some extent (up to 30%). Histamine appears not to be affected by the intact lung but is readily inactivated by slices.

Some vasoactive materials pass through the lung without significant gain or loss of activity. These include epinephrine, prostaglandins A_1 and A_2, angiotensin II, and vasopressin (ADH). More information on the metabolic function of the lung can be found in textbooks of pharmacology.

Several vasoactive and bronchoactive substances are metabolized in the lung and may be released into the circulation under certain conditions. Important among these are the arachidonic acid metabolites (Figure 4.14). Arachidonic acid is formed through the action of the enzyme phospholipase A_2 on phospholipid bound to cell membranes. There are two major synthetic pathways, the initial reactions being catalyzed by the enzymes lipoxygenase and cyclo-

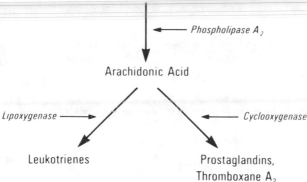

Figure 4.14. Two pathways of arachidonic acid metabolism. The leukotrienes are generated by the lipoxygenase pathway, while the prostaglandins and thromboxane A_2 come from the cyclooxygenase pathway.

oxygenase respectively. The first produces the leukotrienes which include the mediator originally described as slow-reacting substance of anaphylaxis (SRS-A). These compounds cause airway constriction and may have an important role in asthma.‡ Other leukotrienes are involved in inflammatory responses.

The prostaglandins are potent vasoconstrictors or vasodilators. PGE_2 plays an important role in the perinatal period because it helps to constrict the patent ductus arteriosus. Prostaglandins also affect platelet aggregation and are active in other systems such as the kallikrein-kinin clotting cascade. They also may have a role in the bronchoconstriction of asthma.

There is also evidence that the lung plays a role in the clotting mechanism of blood under normal and abnormal conditions. For example, there are large numbers of mast cells containing heparin in the interstitium. Finally, the lung is able to secrete special immunoglobulins, particularly IgA, in the bronchial mucus which contribute to its defenses against infection. The significance of some of these metabolic functions is still obscure but it is clear that the lung has important functions in addition to its main role of gas exchange.

‡ For more details, see JB West: *Pulmonary Pathophysiology—the essentials,* ed 3. Baltimore, Williams & Wilkins, 1987.

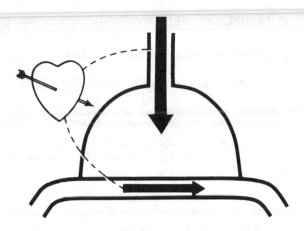

chapter 5

Ventilation-Perfusion Relationships

how matching of gas and blood
determines gas exchange

So far we have considered the movement of air to and from the blood-gas interface, the diffusion of gas across this, and the movement of blood to and from the barrier. It would be natural to assume that if all these processes were adequate, normal gas exchange within the lung would be assured. Unfortunately, this is not so because the matching of ventilation and blood flow within various regions of the lung is critical for adequate gas exchange. Indeed, mismatching of ventilation and blood flow is responsible for most of the defective gas exchange in pulmonary diseases.

In this section we shall look closely at the important (but difficult) subject of how the relations between ventilation and blood flow determine gas exchange. However, first we shall examine two relatively simple causes of impairment of gas exchange, hypoventilation and shunt. Since all these situations result in hypoxemia, that is, an abnormally low P_{O_2} in arterial blood, it is useful to take a preliminary look at normal O_2 transfer.

OXYGEN TRANSPORT FROM AIR TO TISSUES

Figure 5.1 shows how the P_{O_2} falls as the gas moves from the atmosphere in which we live to the mitochondria where it is utilized. The P_{O_2} of air is 20.93% of the total dry gas pressure (that is, excluding water vapor). At sea level, the barometric pressure is 760 mm Hg, and at the body temperature of 37°C, the water vapor pressure of moist inspired gas is 47 mm Hg. Thus, the P_{O_2} of inspired air is $(20.93/100 \times (760 - 47)$ or 149 mm Hg (say 150).

Figure 5.1 is drawn for a hypothetical perfect lung, and it shows that by the time the O_2 has reached the alveoli, the P_{O_2} has fallen to about 100 mm Hg, that is, by one-third. This is because the P_{O_2} of alveolar gas is determined by a balance between two processes: the removal of O_2 by the pulmonary capillary blood on the one hand, and its continual replenishment by alveolar ventilation on the other. (Strictly alveolar ventilation is not continuous but is breath-by-

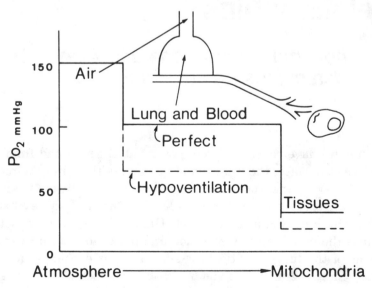

Figure 5.1. Scheme of the O_2 partial pressures from air to tissues. The *solid line* shows a hypothetical perfect situation, and the *dashed line* depicts hypoventilation. Note that hypoventilation depresses the P_{O_2} in the alveolar gas and, therefore, in the tissues.

breath. However, the fluctuation in alveolar P_{O_2} with each breath is only about 3 mm Hg, so the process can be regarded as continuous.) The rate of removal of O_2 from the lung is governed by the O_2 consumption of the tissues and varies little under resting conditions. In practice, therefore, the alveolar P_{O_2} is largely determined by the level of alveolar ventilation. The same applies to the alveolar P_{CO_2}, which is normally about 40 mm Hg.

When the systemic arterial blood reaches the tissue capillaries, O_2 diffuses to the mitochondria, where the P_{O_2} is much lower. The "tissue" P_{O_2} probably differs considerably throughout the body and, in some cells at least, the P_{O_2} is as low as 1 mm Hg. However, the lung is an essential link in the chain of O_2 transport, and any decrease of P_{O_2} in arterial blood must result in a lower tissue P_{O_2}, other things being equal. For the same reasons, impaired pulmonary gas exchange will result in a rise in tissue P_{CO_2}.

HYPOVENTILATION

We have seen that the level of alveolar P_{O_2} is determined by a balance between the rate of removal of O_2 by the blood (which is set by the metabolic demands of the tissues) and the rate of replenishment of O_2 by alveolar ventilation. Thus, if the alveolar ventilation is abnormally low, the alveolar P_{O_2} falls. For similar reasons, the P_{CO_2} rises. This is known as hypoventilation (Figure 5.1).

Causes of hypoventilation include drugs such as morphine and barbiturates which depress the central drive to the respiratory muscles, damage to the chest wall or paralysis of the respiratory muscles, and a high resistance to breathing (for example, very dense gas at great depth underwater). Hypoventilation always causes an increased alveolar and, therefore, arterial P_{CO_2}. The relationship between alveolar ventilation and P_{CO_2} was derived on p. 16:

$$P_{CO_2} = \frac{\dot{V}_{CO_2}}{\dot{V}_A} \times K$$

where $\dot{V}_{CO_2}$ is the CO_2 production, $\dot{V}_A$ is the alveolar ventilation, and K is a constant. This means that if the alveolar ventilation is halved, the P_{CO_2} is doubled, once a steady state has been established.

The relationship between the fall in P_{O_2} and the rise in P_{CO_2} which occurs in hypoventilation can be predicted from the *alveolar gas equation* if we know the composition of inspired gas and the respiratory exchange ratio R. The latter is given by the CO_2 production/O_2

consumption and is determined by the metabolism of the tissues in a steady state. It is sometimes known as the respiratory quotient. A simplified form of the alveolar gas equation is

$$PA_{O_2} = PI_{O_2} - \frac{PA_{CO_2}}{R} + F$$

where F is a small correction factor. This equation shows that if R has its normal value of 0.8, the fall in alveolar P_{O_2} is slightly greater than the rise in P_{CO_2} during hypoventilation. The full version of the equation is given in the Appendix.

Hypoventilation always reduces the alveolar and arterial P_{O_2} except when the subject breathes an enriched O_2 mixture. In this case, the added amount of O_2 per breath can easily make up for the reduced flow of inspired gas.

If alveolar ventilation is suddenly increased (for example, by voluntary hyperventilation), it may take several minutes for the alveolar P_{O_2} and P_{CO_2} to assume their new steady state values. This is because of the O_2 and CO_2 stores in the body. The CO_2 stores are much greater than the O_2 stores because of the large amount of CO_2 in the form of bicarbonate in the blood and interstitial fluid (see Chapter 6). Therefore, the alveolar P_{CO_2} takes longer to come to equilibrium, and during the nonsteady state, the R value of expired gas is high as the CO_2 stores are washed out. Opposite changes occur with hypoventilation.

DIFFUSION

Figure 5.1 shows that in a perfect lung, the P_{O_2} of arterial blood would be the same as that in alveolar gas. In real life, this is not so. One reason is that although the PO_2 of the blood rises closer and closer to that of alveolar gas as the blood traverses the pulmonary capillary (Figure 3.3), it can never quite reach it. Under normal conditions the P_{O_2} difference between alveolar gas and end-capillary blood resulting from incomplete diffusion is immeasurably small but it is shown schematically in Figure 5.2. As we have seen, the difference can become larger when a low O_2 mixture is inspired (Figure 3.3*B*).

SHUNT

Another reason why the P_{O_2} of arterial blood is less than that in alveolar gas is shunted blood. *Shunt* refers to blood which enters the

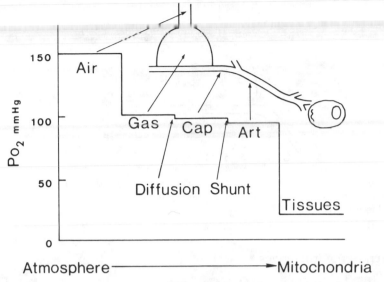

Figure 5.2. Scheme of O_2 transfer from air to tissues showing the depression of arterial P_{O_2} caused by diffusion and shunt. (Modified from JB West: *Ventilation/Blood Flow and Gas Exchange,* ed 4. Oxford, Blackwell, 1985.)

arterial system without going through ventilated areas of lung. In the normal lung, some of the bronchial artery blood is collected by the pulmonary veins after it has perfused the bronchi and its O_2 has been partly depleted. Another source is a small amount of coronary venous blood which drains directly into the cavity of the left ventricle through the Thebesian veins. The effect of the addition of this poorly oxygenated blood is to depress the arterial P_{O_2}. In patients with heart disease, there may be a direct addition of venous blood to arterial blood across a defect between the right and left sides of the heart.

When the shunt is caused by the addition of mixed venous blood (pulmonary arterial) to blood draining from the capillaries (pulmonary venous), it is possible to calculate the amount of the shunt flow (Figure 5.3). The total amount of O_2 leaving the system is the total blood flow $\dot{Q}_T$ multiplied by the O_2 concentration in the arterial blood Ca_{O_2}, or $\dot{Q}_T \times Ca_{O_2}$. This must equal the sum of the amounts of O_2 in the shunted blood, $\dot{Q}_S \times C\bar{v}_{O_2}$, and end-capillary blood, $(\dot{Q}_T - \dot{Q}_S) \times Cc'_{O_2}$. Thus

$$\dot{Q}_T \times Ca_{O_2} = (\dot{Q}_S \times C\bar{v}_{O_2}) + (\dot{Q}_T - \dot{Q}_S) \times Cc'_{O_2}$$

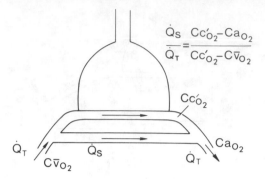

Figure 5.3. Measurement of shunt flow. The oxygen carried in the arterial blood equals the sum of the oxygen carried in the capillary blood and that in the shunted blood (see text).

Rearranging, this gives

$$\frac{\dot{Q}_S}{\dot{Q}_T} = \frac{Cc'_{O_2} - Ca_{O_2}}{Cc'_{O_2} - C\bar{v}_{O_2}}$$

The O_2 concentration of end-capillary blood is usually calculated from the alveolar P_{O_2} and the oxygen dissociation curve (see next chapter).

When the shunt is caused by blood which does not have the same O_2 concentration as mixed venous blood (for example, bronchial vein blood), it is generally not possible to calculate its true magnitude . However, it is often useful to calculate an "as if" shunt, that is, what the shunt *would* be if the observed depression of arterial O_2 concentration was caused by the addition of mixed venous blood.

An important feature of a shunt is that the hypoxemia cannot be abolished by giving the subject 100% O_2 to breathe. This is because the shunted blood that bypasses ventilated alveoli is never exposed to the higher alveolar P_{O_2} so that it continues to depress the arterial P_{O_2}. However, some elevation of the arterial P_{O_2} occurs because of the O_2 added to the capillary blood of ventilated lung. Most of the added O_2 is in the dissolved form, rather than attached to hemoglobin, because the blood that is perfusing ventilated alveoli is nearly fully saturated (see next chapter). Giving the subject 100% O_2 to breathe is a very sensitive measurement of shunt because when the P_{O_2} is high, a small depression of arterial O_2 concentration causes a relatively large fall in P_{O_2} due to the almost flat slope of the O_2 dissociation curve in this region (Figure 5.4).

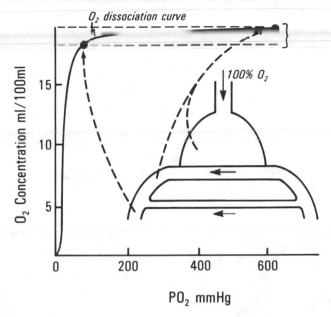

Figure 5.4. Depression of arterial P_{O_2} by shunt during 100% O_2 breathing. The addition of a small amount of shunted blood with its low O_2 concentration greatly reduces the P_{O_2} of arterial blood. This is because the O_2 dissociation curve is so flat when the P_{O_2} is very high.

A shunt usually does not result in a raised P_{CO_2} in arterial blood, even though the shunted blood is rich in CO_2. The reason is that the chemoreceptors sense any elevation of arterial P_{CO_2} and they respond by increasing the ventilation. This reduces the P_{CO_2} of the unshunted blood until the arterial P_{CO_2} is normal. Indeed, in some patients with a shunt, the arterial P_{CO_2} is low because the hypoxemia increases respiratory drive (see Chapter 8).

THE VENTILATION-PERFUSION RATIO

So far we have considered three of the four causes of hypoxemia: hypoventilation, diffusion, and shunt. We now come to the last cause, which is both the commonest and the most difficult to understand, namely, ventilation-perfusion inequality. It turns out that if ventilation and blood flow are mismatched in various regions of the lung, impairment of both O_2 and CO_2 transfer results. The key to understanding how this happens is the ventilation-perfusion ratio.

Consider a model of a lung unit (Figure 2.1) in which the uptake

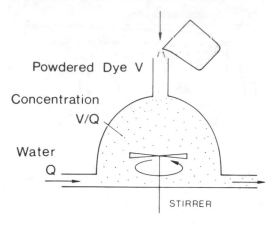

Figure 5.5. Model to illustrate how the ventilation-perfusion ratio determines the P_{O_2} in a lung unit. Powdered dye is added by ventilation at the rate V and removed by blood flow Q to represent the factors controlling alveolar P_{O_2}. The concentration of dye is given by V/Q. (From JB West: *Ventilation/Blood Flow and Gas Exchange,* ed 4. Oxford, Blackwell, 1985.)

of O_2 is being mimicked using dye and water (Figure 5.5). Powdered dye is continuously poured into the unit to represent the addition of O_2 by alveolar ventilation. Water is pumped continuously through the unit to represent the blood flow which removes the O_2. A stirrer mixes the alveolar contents, a process normally accomplished by gaseous diffusion. The key question is: what determines the concentration of dye (or O_2) in the alveolar compartment and, therefore, in the effluent water (or blood)?

It is clear that both the rate at which the dye is added (ventilation) and the rate at which water is pumped (blood flow) will affect the concentration of dye in the model. What may not be intuitively clear is that the concentration of dye is determined by the ratio of these rates. In other words, if dye is added at the rate of V gm/min and water is pumped through at Q liters/min, the concentration of dye in the alveolar compartment and effluent water is V/Q gm/liter.

In exactly the same way, the concentration of O_2 (or better, P_{O_2}) in any lung unit is determined by the ratio of ventilation to blood flow; and not only O_2 but CO_2, N_2, and any other gas that is present under steady state conditions. This is the reason why the ventilation-perfusion ratio plays such a key role in pulmonary gas exchange.

EFFECT OF ALTERING THE VENTILATION-PERFUSION RATIO OF A LUNG UNIT

Let us take a closer look at the way alterations in the ventilation-perfusion ratio of a lung unit affect its gas exchange. Figure 5.6A shows the P_{O_2} and P_{CO_2} in a unit with a normal ventilation-perfusion ratio (about 1). The inspired air has a P_{O_2} of 150 mm Hg (Figure 5.1) and a P_{CO_2} of zero. The mixed venous blood entering the unit has a P_{O_2} of 40 mm Hg and P_{CO_2} of 45 mm Hg. The alveolar P_{O_2} of 100 mm Hg is determined by a balance between the addition of O_2 by ventilation and its removal by blood flow. The normal alveolar P_{CO_2} of 40 mm Hg is set similarly.

Now suppose that the ventilation-perfusion ratio of the unit is gradually reduced by obstructing its ventilation, leaving its blood flow unchanged (Figure 5.6B). It is clear that the O_2 in the unit will fall and the CO_2 will rise, although the relative changes of these two are not immediately obvious.* However, we can easily predict what will eventually happen when the ventilation is completely abolished (ventilation-perfusion ratio of zero). Now the O_2 and CO_2 of alveolar gas and end-capillary blood must be the same as those of mixed venous blood. (In practice, completely obstructed units eventually collapse but we can neglect such long-term effects at the moment.) Note that we are assuming that what happens in one lung unit out of a very large number does not affect the composition of the mixed venous blood.

Suppose instead that the ventilation-perfusion ratio is increased by gradually obstructing blood flow (Figure 5.6C). Now the O_2 rises and the CO_2 falls, eventually reaching the composition of inspired gas when blood flow is abolished (ventilation-perfusion ratio of infinity). Thus, as the ventilation-perfusion ratio of the unit is altered, its gas composition approaches that of mixed venous blood or inspired gas.

A convenient way of depicting these changes is to use the O_2-CO_2 diagram (Figure 5.7). In this, P_{O_2} is plotted on the X axis and P_{CO_2} on

---

*The alveolar gas equation is not applicable here because the respiratory exchange ratio is not constant. The appropriate equation is

$$\frac{\dot{V}_A}{\dot{Q}} = 8.63 \cdot R \cdot \frac{(Ca_{O_2} - C\bar{v}_{O_2})}{Pa_{CO_2}}$$

This is called the ventilation-perfusion ratio equation.

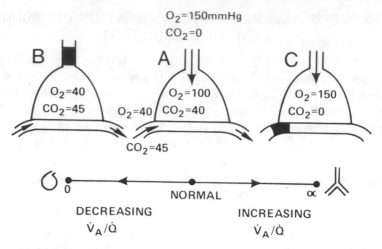

Figure 5.6. Effect of altering the ventilation-perfusion ratio on the P_{O_2} and P_{CO_2} in a lung unit. (From JB West: *Ventilation/Blood Flow and Gas Exchange,* ed 4. Oxford, Blackwell, 1985.)

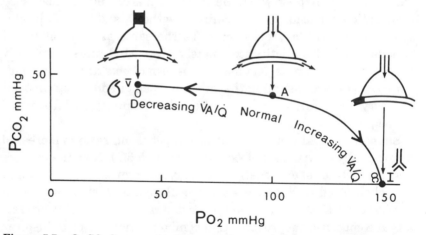

Figure 5.7. O_2-CO_2 diagram showing a ventilation-perfusion ratio line. The P_{O_2} and P_{CO_2} of a lung unit move along this line from the mixed venous point $\bar{v}$ to the inspired gas point I as its ventilation-perfusion ratio is increased (compare Figure 5.6). (From JB West: *Ventilation/Blood Flow and Gas Exchange,* ed 4. Oxford, Blackwell, 1985.)

the Y axis. First, locate the normal alveolar gas composition, point A ($P_{O_2} = 100$, $P_{CO_2} = 40$). If we assume that blood equilibrates with alveolar gas at the end of the capillary (Figures 3.3 and 3.5), this point can equally well represent the end-capillary blood. Next, find the mixed venous point $\bar{v}$ ($P_{O_2} = 40$, $P_{CO_2} = 45$). The bar above v means "mixed" or "mean." Finally, find the inspired point I ($P_{O_2} = 150$,

$P_{CO_2} = 0$). Also, note the similarities between Figures 5.6 and 5.7.

The line jointing $\bar{V}$ to I passing through A shows the changes in alveolar gas (and end-capillary blood) composition that can occur when the ventilation-perfusion ratio is either decreased below normal (A→$\bar{V}$) or increased above normal (A→I). Indeed, this line indicates *all* the possible alveolar gas compositions in a lung which is supplied with gas of composition I and blood of composition $\bar{V}$. For example, such a lung could not contain an alveolus with a P_{O_2} of 70 and P_{CO_2} of 30 mm Hg, since this point does not lie on the ventilation-perfusion line. However, this alveolar composition *could* exist if the mixed venous blood or inspired gas were changed so that the line then passed through this point.

REGIONAL GAS EXCHANGE IN THE LUNG

The way in which the ventilation-perfusion ratio of a lung unit determines its gas exchange can be graphically illustrated by looking at the differences that occur down the upright lung. We saw in Chapters 2 and 4 (Figures 2.7 and 4.8) that ventilation increases slowly from top to bottom of the lung and blood flow increases more rapidly (Figure 5.8). As a consequence, the ventilation-perfusion

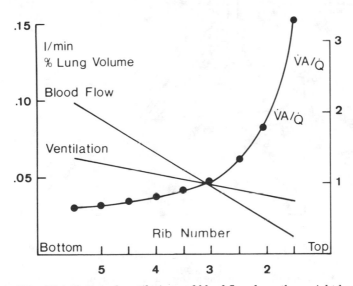

Figure 5.8. Distribution of ventilation and blood flow down the upright lung (compare Figures 2.7 and 4.8). Note that the ventilation-perfusion ratio decreases down the lung. (From JB West: *Ventilation/Blood Flow and Gas Exchange,* ed 4. Oxford, Blackwell, 1985.)

ratio is abnormally high at the top of the lung (where the blood flow is minimal) and much lower at the bottom. We can now use these regional differences in ventilation-perfusion ratio on an O_2-CO_2 diagram (Figure 5.7) to depict the resulting differences in gas exchange.

Figure 5.9 shows the upright lung divided into imaginary horizontal "slices," each of which is located on the ventilation-perfusion line by its own ventilation-perfusion ratio. This ratio is high at the apex so that this point is found toward the right end of the line while the base of the lung is to the left of normal (compare Figure 5.7). It is clear that the P_{O_2} of the alveoli (X axis) decreases markedly down the lung while the P_{CO_2} (Y axis) increases much less.

Figure 5.10 illustrates the values which can be read off a diagram like Figure 5.9. (Of course there will be variations between subjects; the chief aim of this approach is to describe the principles underlying gas exchange.) Note first that the volume of the lung in the slices is less near the apex than the base. Ventilation is less at the top than the bottom, but the differences of blood flow are more marked. Consequently, the ventilation-perfusion ratio decreases down the lung,

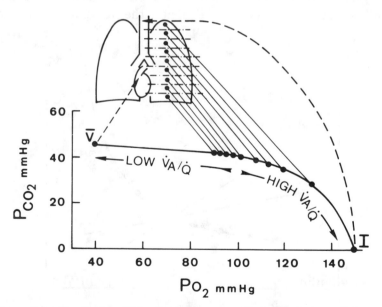

Figure 5.9. Result of combining the pattern of ventilation-perfusion ratio inequality shown in Figure 5.8 with the effects of this on gas exchange as shown in Figure 5.7. Note that the high ventilation-perfusion ratio at the apex results in a high P_{O_2} and low P_{CO_2} there. The opposite is seen at the base. (From JB West: *Ventilation/Blood Flow and Gas Exchange,* ed 4. Oxford, Blackwell, 1985.)

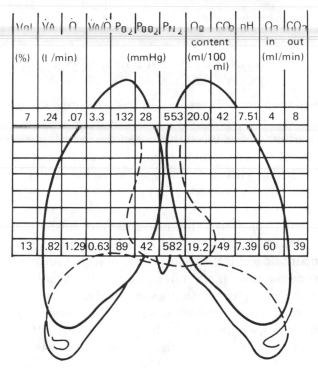

V̇ol (%)	V̇A (l /min)	Q̇	V̇A/Q̇	P_{O_2} (mmHg)	P_{CO_2}	P_{N_2}	O_2 content (ml/100 ml)	CO_2	pH	O_2 in (ml/min)	CO_2 out
7	.24	.07	3.3	132	28	553	20.0	42	7.51	4	8
13	.82	1.29	0.63	89	42	582	19.2	49	7.39	60	39

Figure 5.10. Regional differences in gas exchange down the normal lung. Only the apical and basal values are shown for clarity.

and all the differences in gas exchange follow from this. Note that the P_{O_2} changes by over 40 mm Hg while the difference in P_{CO_2} between apex and base is much less. (Incidentally, the high P_{O_2} at the apex probably accounts for the predilection of adult tuberculosis for this region since it provides a more favorable environment for this organism.) This variation in P_{N_2} is, in effect, by default since the total pressure in the alveolar gas is the same throughout the lung.

The regional differences in P_{O_2} and P_{CO_2} imply differences in the end-capillary contents of these gases which can be obtained from the appropriate dissociation curves (Chapter 6). Note the surprisingly large difference in pH down the lung, which reflects the considerable variation in P_{CO_2} of the blood. The minimal contribution to overall O_2 uptake made by the apex can be mainly attributed to the very low blood flow there. The differences in CO_2 output are much less since this can be shown to be more closely related to ventilation. As a result, the respiratory exchange ratio (CO_2 output/O_2 uptake) is higher at the apex than the base. On exercise, when the distribution of blood flow becomes more uniform, the apex assumes a larger share of the O_2 uptake.

EFFECT OF VENTILATION-PERFUSION INEQUALITY ON OVERALL GAS EXCHANGE

While the regional differences in gas exchange discussed above are of interest, more important to the body as a whole is whether uneven ventilation and blood flow affect the overall gas exchange of the lung, that is, its ability to take up O_2 and put out CO_2. It transpires that a lung with ventilation-perfusion inequality is notable to transfer as much O_2 and CO_2 as a lung that is uniformly ventilated and perfused, other things being equal. Or if the same amounts of gas are being transferred (because these are set by the metabolic demands of the body), the lung with ventilation-perfusion inequality cannot maintain as high an arterial P_{O_2} or as low an arterial P_{CO_2} as a homogeneous lung, again other things being equal.

The reason why a lung with uneven ventilation and blood flow has difficulty oxygenating arterial blood can be illustrated by looking at the differences down the upright lung (Figure 5.11). Here the P_{O_2} at the apex is some 40 mm Hg higher than at the base of the lung. However, the major share of the blood leaving the lung comes from the lower zones, where the P_{O_2} is low. This has the result of depress-

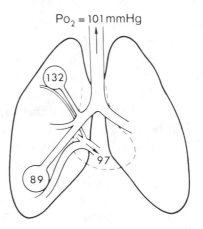

Figure 5.11. Depression of the arterial P_{O_2} by ventilation-perfusion inequality. In this diagram of the upright lung, only two groups of alveoli at the apex and base are shown. The relative sizes of the airways and blood vessels indicate their relative ventilations and blood flows. Because most of the blood comes from the poorly oxygenated base, depression of the blood P_{O_2} is inevitable. (From JB West: *Lancet* 2:1055, 1963.)

ing the arterial P_{O_2}. By contrast, the expired alveolar gas comes more uniformly from apex and base because the differences of ventilation are much less than those for blood flow (Figure 5.8). By the same reasoning, the arterial P_{CO_2} will be elevated since it is higher at the base of the lung than at the apex (Figure 5.10).

An additional reason why uneven ventilation and blood flow depress the arterial P_{O_2} is shown in Figure 5.12. This depicts three groups of alveoli with low, normal, and high ventilation-perfusion ratios. The O_2 concentrations of the effluent blood are 16, 19.5, and 20 ml/100 ml, respectively, and thus the units with the high ventilation-perfusion ratio add relatively little oxygen to the blood, compared with the decrement caused by the alveoli with the low ventilation-perfusion ratio. Thus, the mixed capillary blood has a lower O_2 concentration than that from units with a normal ventilation-perfusion ratio. This can be explained by the nonlinear shape of the oxygen dissociation curve, which means that, although units with a high ventilation-perfusion ratio have a relatively high P_{O_2}, this does not increase the oxygen concentration of their blood very much. This additional reason for the depression of P_{O_2} does not apply to the elevation of the P_{CO_2} since the CO_2 dissociation curve is almost linear in the working range.

The net result of these mechanisms is a depression of the arterial

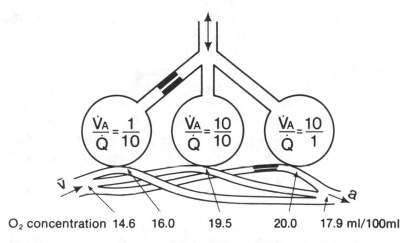

O₂ concentration 14.6   16.0   19.5   20.0   17.9 ml/100ml

Figure 5.12. Additional reason for the depression of arterial P_{O_2} by mismatching of ventilation and blood flow. The lung units with a high ventilation-perfusion ratio add relatively little oxygen to the blood, compared with the decrement caused by alveoli with a low ventilation-perfusion ratio. (Modified from JB West: *Ventilation/Blood Flow and Gas Exchange*, ed 4. Oxford, Blackwell, 1985.)

P_{O_2} below that of the mixed alveolar P_{O_2}—the so-called alveolar-arterial O_2 difference. In the normal upright lung this difference is of trivial magnitude, being only about 4 mm Hg as a result of ventilation-perfusion inequality. Its development is described here only to illustrate how uneven ventilation and blood flow must result in depression of the arterial P_{O_2}. In lung disease, the lowering of arterial P_{O_2} by this mechanism can be extreme.

VENTILATION-PERFUSION INEQUALITY AS A CAUSE OF CO₂ RETENTION

Imagine a lung that is uniformly ventilated and perfused and that is transferring normal amounts of O_2 and CO_2. Suppose that in some magical way, the matching of ventilation and blood flow is suddenly disturbed while everything else remains unchanged. What happens to gas exchange? It transpires that the effect of this "pure" ventilation-perfusion inequality (that is, everything else held constant) is to reduce *both* the O_2 uptake and CO_2 output of the lung. In other words, the lung becomes less efficient as a gas exchanger for both gases. Thus mismatching ventilation and blood flow must cause both hypoxemia and hypercapnia (CO_2 retention), other things being equal.

However, in practice, patients with undoubted ventilation-perfusion inequality often have a normal arterial P_{CO_2}. The reason for this is that whenever the chemoreceptors sense a rising P_{CO_2}, there is an increase in ventilatory drive (Chapter 8). The consequent increase in ventilation to the alveoli usually effectively returns the arterial P_{CO_2} to normal. However, such patients can only maintain a normal P_{CO_2} at the expense of this increased ventilation to their alveoli; the ventilation in excess of what they would normally require is sometimes referred to as *wasted ventilation* and is necessary because the lung units with abnormally high ventilation-perfusion ratios are inefficient at eliminating CO_2. Such units are said to constitute an *alveolar dead space*.

While the increase in ventilation to a lung with ventilation-perfusion inequality is usually effective at reducing the arterial P_{CO_2}, it is much less effective at increasing the arterial P_{O_2}. The reason for the different behavior of the two gases lies in the shapes of the CO_2 and O_2 dissociation curves (Chapter 6). The CO_2 dissociation curve is almost straight in the physiological range, with the result that an increase in ventilation will raise the CO_2 output of lung units with both high and low ventilation-perfusion ratios. By contrast, the almost flat top of the O_2 dissociation curve means that only units with moderately low ventilation-perfusion ratios will benefit appreciably from the increased ventilation. Those units which are very high on the dissociation curve (high ventilation-perfusion ratio) increase the O_2 concentration of their effluent blood very little (Figure 5.12). Those units which have a very low ventilation-perfusion ratio continue to put out blood which has an O_2 concentration close to that of mixed venous blood. The net result is that the mixed arterial P_{O_2} rises only modestly, and some hypoxemia always remains.

MEASUREMENT OF VENTILATION-PERFUSION INEQUALITY

How can we asses the amount of ventilation-perfusion inequality in a lung? Radioactive gases can be used to define topographical differences in ventilation and blood flow in the upright normal lung (Figures 2.7 and 4.8), but in most circumstances significant inequality exists between closely adjacent units, and this cannot be distinguished by counters over the chest. In practice, we turn to indices based on the resulting impairment of gas exchange.†

One useful measurement is the *alveolar-arterial* P_{O_2} *difference*. This is obtained by subtracting the arterial P_{O_2} from the so-called "ideal" alveolar P_{O_2}. The latter is the P_{O_2} which the lung *would* have if there were no ventilation-perfusion inequality and it was exchanging gas at the same respiratory exchange ratio as the real lung. It is derived from the alveolar gas equation.

$$PA_{O_2} = PI_{O_2} - \frac{PA_{CO_2}}{R} + F$$

The arterial P_{CO_2} is used for the alveolar value.

An increased alveolar-arterial O_2 difference is caused both by abnormally low and abnormally high ventilation-perfusion ratios within the lung, though chiefly the former. It is possible to separately assess the approximate contribution of these two groups to the impairment of gas exchange. For the effect of the units with low ventilation-perfusion ratios we can calculate the *physiologic shunt*. To do this we pretend that all the hypoxemia is caused by blood

---

† For more details of this difficult subject, see JB West: *Pulmonary Pathophysiology—the essentials,* ed 3. Baltimore, Williams & Wilkins, 1987.

passing through unventilated alveoli (although we know this is an oversimplification). The shunt equation is then used in the form

$$\frac{\dot{Q}_{PS}}{\dot{Q}_t} = \frac{Ci_{O_2} - Ca_{O_2}}{Ci_2 - C\bar{v}_{O_2}}$$

where $\dot{Q}_{PS}$ refers to physiologic shunt and Ci_{O_2} means the O_2 content of blood draining from "ideal" alveoli. The latter is found from the ideal alveolar P_{O_2} and the O_2 dissociation curve.

The effect of lung units with abnormally high ventilation-perfusion ratios is assessed by calculating the *physiologic dead space*. Here we pretend that all the lowering of P_{CO_2} in expired gas is caused by unperfused alveoli together with the anatomic dead space. We use the Bohr dead space equation in the form

$$\frac{V_{D_{phys}}}{V_T} = \frac{Pa_{CO_2} - P_{E_{CO_2}}}{Pa_{CO_2}}$$

where $V_{D_{phys}}$ refers to physiologic dead space. Most patients with chronic obstructive lung disease, for example, have increases in both the physiologic shunt and dead space.

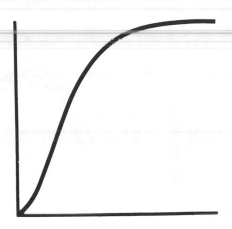

chapter 6

Gas Transport to the Periphery

how gases are moved to the peripheral tissues

OXYGEN

O_2 is carried in the blood in two forms—dissolved and in combination with hemoglobin.

Dissolved O_2

This obeys Henry's law, that is, the amount dissolved is proportional to the partial pressure (Figure 6.1). For each mm Hg of P_{O_2}, there is 0.003 ml O_2/100 ml of blood (sometimes written 0.003 vol %). Thus, normal arterial blood with a P_{O_2} of 100 mm Hg contains 0.3 ml O_2/100 ml.

It is easy to see that this way of transporting O_2 must be inadequate for man. Suppose that the O_2 consumption during strenuous

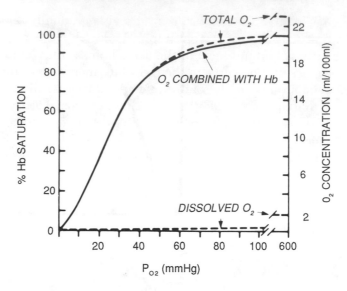

Figure 6.1. O_2 dissociation curve (*solid line*) for pH 7.4, P_{CO_2} 40 mm Hg, and 37°C. The total blood O_2 concentration is also shown for a hemoglobin concentration of 15 gm/100 ml of blood.

exercise is 3,000 ml/min and that all the O_2 is extracted from arterial blood by the peripheral tissues. Then, since cardiac output, O_2 consumption, and the arterial-venous O_2 difference are related by the Fick principle (p. 39),

$$\dot{Q} = \frac{\dot{V}_{O_2}}{Ca_{O_2} - C\bar{v}_{O_2}}$$

then

$$\dot{Q} = \frac{3000}{0.003 - 0} \text{ where } Ca_{O_2} = 0.003 \text{ ml/ml}$$

$$= 1,000,000 \text{ ml/min or } 1000 \text{ liter/min!}$$

Clearly, an additional method of transporting O_2 is required.

Hemoglobin

Heme is an iron-porphyrin compound and this is joined to the protein globin, which consists of four polypeptide chains. The chains are of two types, alpha and beta, and differences in their amino acid sequences give rise to various types of human hemoglobin. Normal adult hemoglobin is known as A. Hemoglobin F (fetal) makes up part of the hemoglobin of the newborn infant and is gradually replaced over the first year or so of postnatal life. Hemoglobin S (sickle) has valine instead of glutamic acid in the beta chains. This results in a shift in the dissociation curve to the right but, more important, the deoxygenated form is poorly soluble and crystallizes within the red cell. As a consequence the cell shape changes from biconcave to crescent or sickle shaped with increased fragility and a tendency to thrombus formation. Many other varieties of hemoglobin have now been described, some with bizarre O_2 affinities. For more information about hemoglobin, consult a textbook of biochemistry.

Normal hemoglobin A can have its ferrous ion oxidized to the ferric form by various drugs and chemicals, including nitrites, sulfonamides, and acetanilid. This ferric form is known as methemoglobin. There is a congenital cause in which the enzyme methemoglobin reductase is deficient within the red blood cell. Another abnormal form is sulfhemoglobin. These compounds are not useful for O_2 carriage.

O_2 Dissociation Curve

O_2 forms an easily reversible combination with hemoglobin (Hb) to give oxyhemoglobin: $O_2 + Hb \rightleftharpoons HbO_2$. Suppose we take a number of glass containers (tonometers), each containing a small volume of blood, and add gas with various concentrations of O_2. After allowing time for the gas and blood to reach equilibrium, we measure the P_{O_2} of the gas and the O_2 content of the blood. Knowing that 0.003 ml O_2 will be dissolved in each 100 ml of blood/mm Hg P_{O_2}, we can calculate the O_2 combined with Hb (Figure 6.1). Note that the amount of O_2 carried by the Hb increases rapidly up to a P_{O_2} of about 50 mm Hg, but above that the curve becomes much flatter. The maximum amount of O_2 that can be combined with Hb is called the O_2 *capacity*. It can be measured by exposing the blood to a very high P_{O_2} (say 600 mm Hg) and subtracting the dissolved O_2. One gram of pure Hb can combine with 1.39* ml O_2, and since normal blood has about 15 gm of Hb/100 ml, the O_2 capacity is about 20.8 ml O_2/100 ml of blood.

The O_2 *saturation* of Hb is given by

$$\frac{O_2 \text{ combined with Hb}}{O_2 \text{ capacity}} \times 100$$

---

*Some measurements give 1.34 or 1.36 ml. The reason is that under the normal conditions of the body, some of the hemoglobin is in forms such as methemoglobin that cannot combine with O_2.

The O_2 saturation of arterial blood with P_{O_2} of 100 mm Hg is about 97.5% while that of mixed venous blood with a P_{O_2} of 40 mm Hg is about 75%. It is important to grasp the relationships between P_{O_2}, O_2 saturation, and O_2 concentration (Figure 6.2). For example, suppose a severely anemic patient with a Hb concentration of only 10 gm/100 ml of blood has normal lungs and an arterial P_{O_2} of 100 mm Hg. His O_2 capacity will be $20.8 \times 10/15 = 13.9$ ml/100 ml. His O_2 saturation will be 97.5% (at normal pH, P_{CO_2}, and temperature), but the O_2 combined with Hb will be only 13.5 ml/100 ml. Dissolved O_2 will contribute 0.3 ml, giving a total O_2 concentration of 13.8 ml/100 ml of blood. In general the oxygen content (or concentration) of blood (in ml O_2/100 ml blood) is given by:

$$\left(1.39 \times Hb \times \frac{Sat}{100}\right) + 0.003\ P_{O_2}$$

where Hb is the hemoglobin concentration in gm/100 ml, Sat is the percentage saturation of the hemoglobin, and P_{O_2} is in mm Hg.

The curved shape of the O_2 dissociation curve has several physiological advantages. The flat upper portion means that even if the P_{O_2} in alveolar gas falls somewhat, loading of O_2 will be little affected. In addition, as the red cell takes up O_2 along the pulmonary capillary (Figure 3.3), a large partial pressure difference between alveolar gas and blood continues to exist even when most of the O_2 has been transferred. As a result the diffusion process is hastened. The steep

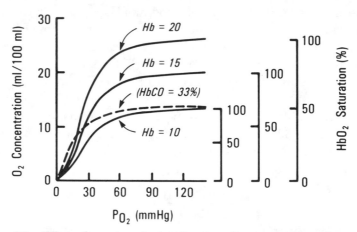

Figure 6.2. Effects of anemia and polycythemia on O_2 concentration and saturation. In addition, the *broken line* shows the O_2 dissociation curve when one-third of the normal hemoglobin is bound to CO. Note that the curve is shifted to the left.

lower part of the dissociation curve means that the peripheral tissues can withdraw large amounts of O_2 for only a small drop in capillary P_{O_2}. This maintenance of blood P_{O_2} assists the diffusion of O_2 into the tissue cells.

Because reduced Hb is purple, a low arterial O_2 saturation causes *cyanosis*. However, this is not a reliable sign of mild desaturation because its recognition depends on so many variables, such as lighting conditions and skin pigmentation. Since it is the amount of reduced Hb that is important, cyanosis is often marked when polycythemia is present but is difficult to detect in anemic patients.

The O_2 dissociation curve is shifted to the right by an increase in H^+ concentration, P_{CO_2}, temperature, and the concentration of 2,3-diphosphoglycerate in the red cells (Figure 6.3). Opposite changes shift it to the left. Most of the effect of P_{CO_2}, which is known as the *Bohr effect,* can be attributed to its action on H^+ concentration. A rightward shift means more unloading of O_2 at a given P_{O_2} in a tissue capillary. A simple way to remember these shifts is that an

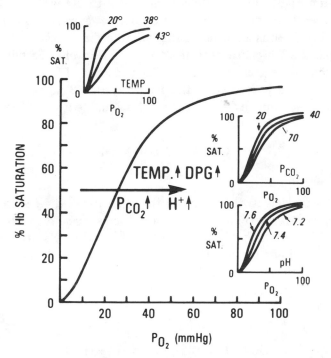

Figure 6.3. Rightward shift of the O_2 dissociation curve by increase of H^+, P_{CO_2}, temperature, and 2,3-diphosphoglycerate (*DPG*).

exercising muscle is acid, hypercarbic, and hot, and it benefits from increased unloading of O_2 from its capillaries.

The environment of the Hb within the red cell also affects the O_2 dissociation curve. An increase in 2,3-diphosphoglycerate (DPG), which is an end-product of red cell metabolism, shifts the curve to the right. An increase in concentration of this material occurs in chronic hypoxia, for example, at high altitude or in the presence of chronic lung disease. As a result, the unloading of O_2 to peripheral tissues is assisted. A useful measure of the position of the dissociation curve is the P_{O_2} for 50% O_2 saturation (P_{50}). The normal value for human blood is about 27 mm Hg.

Carbon monoxide interferes with the O_2 transport function of blood by combining with Hb to form carboxyhemoglobin (COHb). CO has about 240 times the affinity of O_2 for Hb; this means that CO will combine with the same amount of Hb as O_2 when the CO partial pressure is 240 times lower. In fact the CO dissociation curve is almost identical in shape to the O_2 dissociation curve of Figure 6.3, except that the Pco axis is greatly compressed. For example, at a Pco of 0.16 mm Hg, 75% of the Hb is combined with CO as COHb. For this reason small amounts of CO can tie up a large proportion of the Hb in the blood, thus making it unavailable for O_2 carriage. If this happens, the Hb concentration of P_{O_2} of blood may be normal but its O_2 content is grossly reduced. The presence of COHb also shifts the O_2 dissociation curve to the left (Figure 6.2), thus interfering with the unloading of O_2. This is an additional feature of the toxicity of CO.

CARBON DIOXIDE

CO_2 Carriage

CO_2 is carried in the blood in three forms—dissolved, as bicarbonate, and in combination with proteins as carbamino compounds (Figure 6.4). *Dissolved* CO_2, like O_2, obeys Henry's law, but CO_2 is some 20 times more soluble than O_2. As a result dissolved CO_2 plays a significant role in its carriage in that about 10% of the gas that is evolved into the lung from the blood is in the dissolved form (Figure 6.5).

Bicarbonate is formed in blood by the following sequence:

$$CO_2 + H_2O \overset{CA}{\rightleftharpoons} H_2CO_3 \rightleftharpoons H^+ + HCO_3^-$$

The first reaction is very slow in plasma but fast within the red blood cell because of the presence there of the enzyme *carbonic anhydrase*

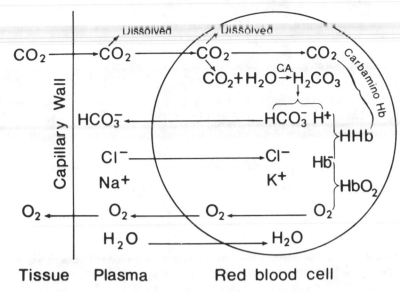

Figure 6.4. Scheme of the uptake of CO_2 and liberation of O_2 in systemic capillaries. Exactly opposite events occur in the pulmonary capillaries.

(CA). The second reaction, ionic dissociation of carbonic acid, is fast without an enzyme. When the concentration of these ions rises within the red cell, HCO_3^- diffuses out but H^+ cannot easily do this because the cell membrane is relatively impermeable to cations. Thus, in order to maintain electrical neutrality, Cl^- ions diffuse into the cell from the plasma, the so-called *chloride shift* (Figure 6.4). The movement of chloride is in accordance with the Gibbs-Donnan equilibrium.

Some of the H^+ ions liberated are bound to hemoglobin

$$H^+ + HbO_2 \rightleftharpoons H^+ \cdot Hb + O_2$$

This occurs because reduced Hb is less acid (that is, a better proton acceptor) than the oxygenated form. Thus, the presence of reduced Hb in the peripheral blood helps with the loading of CO_2 while the oxygenation which occurs in the pulmonary capillary assists in the unloading. The fact that the deoxygenation of the blood increases its ability to carry CO_2 is often known as the *Haldane effect*.

These events associated with the uptake of CO_2 by blood increase the osmolar content of the red cell and, consequently, water enters the cell, thus increasing its volume. When the cells pass through the lung, they shrink a little.

Carbamino compounds are formed by the combination of CO_2 with

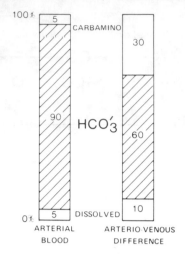

Figure 6.5. The *first column* shows the proportions of the total CO_2 concentration in arterial blood. The *second column* shows the proportions which make up the arterial-venous difference.

terminal amine groups in blood proteins. The most important protein is the globin of hemoglobin: $Hb \cdot NH_2 + CO_2 \rightleftharpoons Hb \cdot NH \cdot COOH$, giving carbamino-hemoglobin. This reaction occurs rapidly without an enzyme, and reduced Hb can bind more CO_2 as carbamino-hemoglobin than HbO_2. Thus, again unloading of O_2 in peripheral capillaries facilitates the loading of CO_2 while oxygenation has the opposite effect.

The relative contributions of the various forms of CO_2 in blood to the total CO_2 content are shown in Figure 6.5. Note that the great bulk of the CO_2 is in the form of bicarbonate. The amount dissolved is small as is that in the form of carbamino-hemoglobin. However, these proportions do not reflect the changes that take place when CO_2 is loaded or unloaded by the blood. Of the total venous-arterial difference, about 60% is attributable to HCO_3^-, 30% to carbamino compounds, and 10% to dissolved CO_2.

CO_2 Dissociation Curve

The relationship between the P_{CO_2} and the total CO_2 concentration of blood is shown in Figure 6.6. Note that the CO_2 dissociation curve is much more linear than the O_2 dissociation curve (Figure 6.1). Note also that the lower the saturation of Hb with O_2, the larger the CO_2 concentration for a given P_{CO_2}. As we have seen, this *Haldane effect* can be explained by the better ability of reduced Hb to mop up the H^+ ions produced when carbonic acid dissociates, and the greater

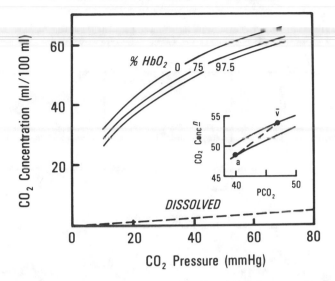

Figure 6.6. CO_2 dissociation curves for blood of different O_2 saturations. Note that oxygenated blood carries less CO_2 for the same P_{CO_2}. The *inset* shows the "physiological" curve between arterial and mixed venous blood.

facility of reduced Hb to form carbamino-hemoglobin. Figure 6.7A shows that the CO_2 dissociation curve is considerably steeper than that for O_2. For example, in the range of 40–50 mm Hg, the CO_2 concentration changes by about 4.7, compared with an O_2 concentration of only about 1.7 ml/100 ml.

A useful way of displaying the interactions between the O_2 and CO_2 dissociation curves is by means of the O_2-CO_2 diagram (compare Figures 5.7 and 5.9). Figure 6.7B shows that the lines of equal O_2 and CO_2 concentration are not straight and parallel to the axes as they would be if the concentrations were simply proportional to the partial pressures. Choose a P_{O_2} on the X axis (say, 50 mm Hg). Follow this P_{O_2} vertically (increasing P_{CO_2}) and lines of decreasing O_2 concentration will be encountered (Bohr effect). The same procedure following a given P_{CO_2} to the right (increasing P_{O_2}) will give decreasing CO_2 concentrations (Haldane effect). Such a diagram was used to read off the O_2 and CO_2 concentrations shown in Figure 5.10 from the O_2-CO_2 diagram of Figure 5.9.

ACID-BASE STATUS

The transport of CO_2 has a profound effect on the acid-base status of blood and the body as a whole. The lung excretes over 10,000 mEq of carbonic acid per day compared with less than 100 mEq of fixed

A

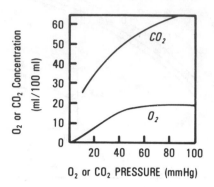

B

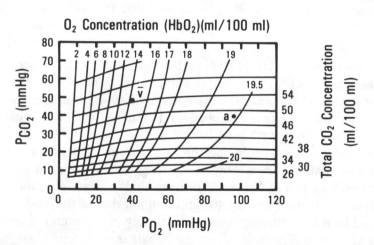

Figure 6.7. (A) Typical O_2 and CO_2 dissociation curves plotted with the same scales. Note that the CO_2 curve is much steeper. (B) O_2-CO_2 diagram showing lines of equal O_2 and CO_2 concentration. The lines are not parallel to the X and Y axes because of the Bohr and Haldane effects. Typical arterial (a) and mixed venous ($\bar{v}$) points are shown.

acids by the kidney. Therefore, by altering alveolar ventilation and thus the elimination of CO_2, the body has great control over its acid-base balance. This subject will be treated only briefly here because it overlaps the area of renal physiology.

The pH resulting from the solution of CO_2 in blood and the consequent dissociation of carbonic acid is given by the Henderson-Hasselbalch equation. It is derived as follows. In the equation

$$H_2CO_3 \rightleftharpoons H^+ + HCO_3^-$$

the law of the mass action gives the dissociation constant of carbonic acid K_A' as

$$\frac{(H^+) \times (HCO_3^-)}{(H_2CO_3)}$$

Now, since the concentration of carbonic acid is proportional to the concentration of dissolved carbon dioxide, we can change the constant and write

$$K_A = \frac{(H^+) \times (HCO_3^-)}{(CO_2)}$$

Taking logarithms

$$\log K_A = \log (H^+) + \log \frac{(HCO_3^-)}{(CO_2)}$$

whence

$$-\log (H^+) = -\log K_A + \log \frac{(HCO_3^-)}{(CO_2)}$$

Since pH is the negative logarithm

$$pH = pK_A + \log \frac{(HCO_3^-)}{(CO_2)}$$

Because CO_2 obeys Henry's law, the CO_2 concentration (in mM/liter) can be replaced by $(P_{CO_2} \times 0.03)$. The equation then becomes

$$pH = pK_A + \log \frac{(HCO_3^-)}{0.03\,P_{CO_2}}$$

The value of pK_A is 6.1, and the normal HCO_3^- concentration in arterial blood is 24 mM/liter. Substituting gives

$$pH = 6.1 + \log \frac{24}{0.03 \times 40}$$

$$= 6.1 + \log 20$$

$$= 6.1 + 1.3$$

Therefore,   pH = 7.4.

Note that as long as the ratio of bicarbonate concentration to $(P_{O_2} \times 0.03)$ remains equal to 20, the pH will remain at 7.4. The bicarbonate concentration is determined chiefly by the kidney and the P_{CO_2} by the lung.

The relationships between pH, P_{CO_2}, and HCO_3^- are conveniently shown on a Davenport diagram (Figure 6.8). The two axes show HCO_3^- and pH, and lines of equal P_{CO_2} sweep across the diagram. Normal plasma is represented by point A. The line CAB shows the relationship between HCO_3^- and pH as carbonic acid is added to whole blood, that is, it is part of the titration curve for blood and is called the *buffer line*. The slope of this line is steeper than that observed for plasma separated from blood because of the presence of hemoglobin, which has a buffering action. The slope of the line measured on whole blood *in vitro* is usually a little different from that found in a patient because of the buffering action of the interstitial fluid and other body tissues.

Another way of portraying these relationships is shown in Figure 6.9 where log P_{CO_2} is plotted against pH. On this diagram, straight lines of equal HCO_3^- concentrations run from top left to bottom right and intercept the horizontal $P_{CO_2} = 40$ mm Hg line as shown. The normal buffer line is also straight and somewhat steeper than the HCO_3^- lines. In addition, a base excess scale is shown on the curved line (see below). The pH-log P_{CO_2} diagram is often used in clinical assessment of acid-base disturbances. It gives essentially the same information as the pH-bicarbonate diagram, but it has the advantage that the points can be more easily plotted in practice since the pH and P_{CO_2} can be quickly measured on a single blood sample by means of blood gas electrodes. Once the Davenport diagram has been mastered, the pH-log P_{CO_2} diagram can be easily used.

The ratio of bicarbonate to P_{CO_2} can be disturbed in four ways: the P_{CO_2} can be raised or lowered, and the bicarbonate also. Each of these four disturbances gives rise to a characteristic acid-base change.

Respiratory Acidosis

This is caused by an increase in P_{CO_2} which reduces the HCO_3^-/P_{CO_2} ratio and thus depresses the pH. This corresponds to a movement from A to B in Figure 6.8 (or Figure 6.9). Whenever the P_{CO_2} rises, the bicarbonate must also increase to some extent because of dissociation of the carbonic acid produced. This is reflected by the left up-

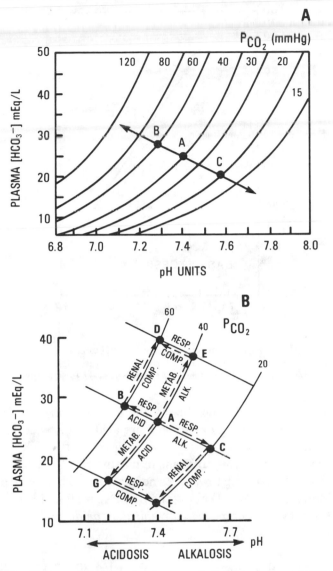

Figure 6.8. Davenport diagram showing the relationships between HCO_3^-, pH, and P_{CO_2}. A shows the buffer line BAC. B shows the changes occurring in respiratory and metabolic acidosis and alkalosis (see text).

ward slope of the blood buffer line in Figure 6.8. However, the ratio HCO_3^-/P_{CO_2} falls. CO_2 retention can be caused by hypoventilation (p. 53) or ventilation-perfusion inequality.

If respiratory acidosis persists, the kidney responds by conserving

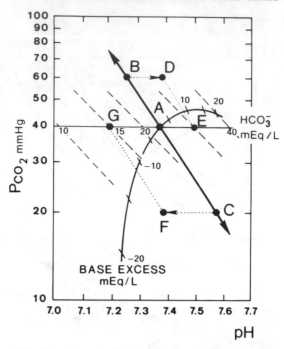

Figure 6.9.   pH-log P_{CO_2} diagram showing the normal buffer line and the base excess scale. The *lettered points* correspond to those in Figure 6.8. (Modified from O Siggaard-Andersen and K Engel: *Scand J Clin Lab Invest* 12:177, 1960.)

HCO_3^-. It is prompted to do this by the increased P_{CO_2} in the renal tubular cells, which then excrete a more acid urine by secreting H^+ ions. The H^+ ions are excreted as $H_2PO_4^-$ or NH_4^+; the HCO_3^- ions are reabsorbed. The resulting increase in plasma HCO_3^- then moves the HCO_3^-/P_{CO_2} ratio back up toward its normal level. This corresponds to the movement from B to D along the line $P_{CO_2} = 60$ mm Hg in Figure 6.8 and is known as *compensated respiratory acidosis*. Typical events would be

$$pH = 6.1 + \log \frac{24}{0.03 \times 40} = 6.1 + \log 20 = 7.4 \qquad \text{(Normal)}$$

$$pH = 6.1 + \log \frac{28}{0.03 \times 60} = 6.1 + \log 15.6 = 7.29$$

$$\text{(Respiratory acidosis)}$$

$$ph = 6.1 + \log \frac{33}{0.03 \times 60} = 6.1 + \log 18.3 = 7.36$$

$$\text{(Compensated respiratory acidosis)}$$

The renal compensation is rarely complete and so the pH does not fully return to its normal level of 7.4. The extent of the renal compensation can be determined from the *base excess*. This is the vertical distance between the buffer lines BA and DE. Alternatively, the base excess can be read off the curved scale on Figure 6.9 by drawing a line through the blood point parallel to the buffer line and noting its intersection with the scale.

Respiratory Alkalosis

This is caused by a decrease in P_{CO_2} which increases the HCO_3^-/P_{CO_2} ratio and thus elevates the pH (movement from A to C in Figure 6.8). A decrease in P_{CO_2} is caused by hyperventilation, for example, at high altitude (see Chapter 9). Renal compensation occurs by an increased excretion of bicarbonate, thus returning the HCO_3^-/P_{CO_2} ratio back toward normal (C to F along the line $P_{CO_2} = 20$ mm Hg). After a prolonged stay at high altitude, the renal compensation may be nearly complete. There is a negative base excess, or a *base deficit*.

Metabolic Acidosis

In this context "metabolic" means a primary change in HCO_3^-, that is, the numerator of the Henderson-Hasselbalch equation. In metabolic acidosis, the ratio of HCO_3^- to P_{CO_2} falls, thus depressing the pH. The HCO_3^- may be lowered by the accumulation of acids in the blood, as in uncontrolled diabetes mellitus, or following tissue hypoxia which releases lactic acid. The corresponding change in Figure 6.8 is a movement from A toward G.

In this instance, respiratory compensation occurs by an increase in ventilation which lowers the P_{CO_2} and raises the depressed HCO_3^-/P_{CO_2} ratio. The stimulus to raise the ventilation is chiefly the action of H^+ ions on the peripheral chemoreceptors (Chapter 8). In Figure 6.8, the point moves in the direction G to F (although not as far as F). There is a base deficit or negative base excess.

Metabolic Alkalosis

Here an increase in HCO_3^- raises the HCO_3^-/P_{CO_2} ratio and, thus, the pH. Excessive ingestion of alkalis and loss of acid gastric juice are causes. In Figure 6.8, the movement is in the direction A to E. Respiratory compensation sometimes occurs by a reduction in alveolar ventilation which raises the P_{CO_2}. Point E then moves in the direction of D (although not all the way). However, respiratory compensation in metabolic alkalosis is often small and may be absent. Base excess is increased.

It should be noted that mixed respiratory and metabolic disturbances often occur, and it may then be difficult to unravel the sequence of events.

BLOOD-TISSUE GAS EXCHANGE

O_2 and CO_2 move between the systemic capillary blood and the tissue cells by simple diffusion, just as they move between the capillary blood and alveolar gas in the lung. We saw in Chapter 3 that the rate of transfer of gas through a tissue sheet is proportional to the tissue area and the difference in gas partial pressure between the two sides, and inversely proportional to the thickness. The thickness of the blood-gas barrier is less than 0.5 micron, but the distance between open capillaries in resting muscle is on the order of 50 microns. During exercise when the O_2 consumption of the muscle increases, additional capillaries open up, thus reducing the diffusion distance and increasing the area for diffusion. Because CO_2 diffuses about 20 times faster than O_2 through tissue (Figure 3.1), elimination of CO_2 is much less of a problem than O_2 delivery.

The way in which the P_{O_2} falls in tissue between adjacent open capillaries is shown schematically in Figure 6.10. As the O_2 diffuses away from the capillary, it is consumed by tissue, and the P_{O_2} falls. In A the balance between O_2 consumption and delivery (determined by the capillary P_{O_2} and the intercapillary distance) results in an adequate P_{O_2} in all the tissue. In B, the intercapillary distance or the O_2 consumption has been increased until the P_{O_2} at one point in the tissue falls to zero. This is referred to as a *critical* situation. In C there is an anoxic region where aerobic (that is, O_2 utilizing) metab-

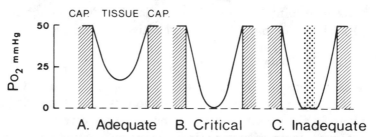

Figure 6.10. Scheme showing the fall in P_{O_2} between adjacent open capillaries. In A, oxygen delivery is adequate; in B, critical, and in C, inadequate for aerobic metabolism in the central core of tissue.

olism is impossible. Under these conditions, the tissue turns to anaerobic glycolysis with the formation of lactic acid.

How low can the tissue P_{O_2} fall before O_2 utilization ceases? In measurements on suspensions of liver mitochondria *in vitro*, O_2 consumption continues at the same rate until the P_{O_2} falls to the region of 3 mm Hg. Thus, it appears that the purpose of the much higher P_{O_2} in capillary blood is to ensure an adequate pressure for diffusion of O_2 to the mitochondria and that at the sites of O_2 utilization the P_{O_2} may be very low.

An inadequate supply of O_2 to tissues is called tissue hypoxia. It can be due to (1) a low P_{O_2} in arterial blood caused, for example, by pulmonary disease ("hypoxic hypoxia"); (2) a reduced ability of blood to carry O_2 as in anemia or carbon monoxide poisoning ("anemic hypoxia"); or (3) a reduction in tissue blood flow, either generalized, as in shock, or because of local obstruction ("circulatory hypoxia"). A fourth cause is some toxic substance which interferes with the ability of the tissues to utilize available O_2 ("histotoxic hypoxia"). An example is cyanide, which prevents the use of O_2 by cytochrome oxidase. In this case, the O_2 concentrations of both arterial and venous blood may be high, and the O_2 consumption of the tissue extremely low since these are related by the Fick principle as applied to peripheral O_2 consumption.

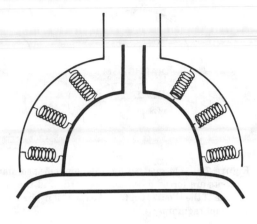

chapter 7

Mechanics of Breathing

how the lung is supported and moved

We saw in Chapter 2 that gas gets to and from the alveoli by the process of ventilation. The present chapter deals with the forces that move the lung and chest wall and the resistances they overcome.

MUSCLES OF RESPIRATION

Inspiration

The most important muscle of inspiration is the *diaphragm*. This consists of a thin, dome-shaped sheet of muscle which is inserted into the lower ribs. It is supplied by the phrenic nerves from cervical segments 3, 4, and 5. When it contracts, the abdominal contents are forced downward and forward, and the vertical dimension of the chest cavity is increased. In addition, the rib margins are lifted and moved out, causing an increase in the transverse diameter of the thorax (Figure 7.1).

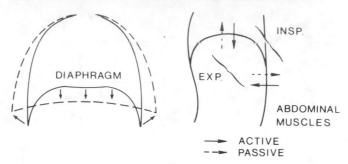

Figure 7.1. On inspiration, the dome-shaped diaphragm contracts, the abdominal contents are forced down and forward, and the rib cage is lifted. Both increase the volume of the thorax. On forced expiration, the abdominal muscles contract and push the diaphragm up.

In normal tidal breathing, the level of the diaphragm moves about 1 cm or so, but on forced inspiration and expiration, a total excursion of up to 10 cm may occur. When the diaphragm is paralyzed, it moves *up* rather than *down* with inspiration because the intrathoracic pressure falls. This is known as *paradoxical movement* and can be demonstrated at fluoroscopy when the subject sniffs.

The *external intercostal muscles* connect adjacent ribs and slope downward and forward (Figure 7.2). When they contract, the ribs are pulled upward and forward, causing an increase in both the lateral and anteroposterior diameters of the thorax. The lateral dimension increases because of the "bucket-handle" movement of the ribs. The intercostal muscles are supplied by intercostal nerves which come off the spinal cord at the same level. Paralysis of the intercostal muscles alone does not seriously affect breathing because the diaphragm is so effective.

The *accessory muscles of inspiration* include the scalene muscles which elevate the first two ribs, and the sternomastoids which raise the sternum. There is little if any activity in these muscles during quiet breathing, but during exercise they may contract vigorously. Other muscles which play a minor role include the alae nasi, which cause flaring of the nostrils, and small muscles in the neck and head.

Expiration

This is passive during quiet breathing. The lung and chest wall are elastic and tend to return to their equilibrium positions after being actively expanded during inspiration. During exercise and voluntary hyperventilation, expiration becomes active. The most

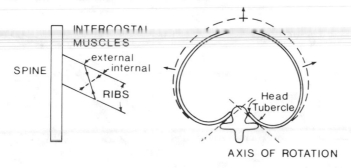

Figure 7.2. When the external intercostal muscles contract, the ribs are pulled upward and forward, and they rotate on an axis joining the tubercle and head of rib. As a result, both the lateral and anteroposterior diameters of the thorax increase. The internal intercostals have the opposite action.

important muscles of expiration are those of the *abdominal wall,* including the rectus abdominus, internal and external oblique muscles, and transversus abdominus. When these muscles contract, intra-abdominal pressure is raised, and the diaphragm is pushed upward. They also contract forcefully during coughing, vomiting, and defecation.

The *internal intercostal muscles* assist active expiration by pulling the ribs downward and inward (opposite to the action of the external intercostal muscles), thus decreasing the thoracic volume. In addition, they stiffen the intercostal spaces to prevent them from bulging outward during straining. Recent studies show that the actions of the respiratory muscles, especially the intercostals, are more complicated than this brief account suggests.

ELASTIC PROPERTIES OF THE LUNG

Pressure-Volume Curve

Suppose we take an excised dog lung, cannulate the trachea, and place it inside a jar (Figure 7.3). When the pressure within the jar is reduced below atmospheric pressure the lung expands and its change in volume can be measured with a spirometer. The pressure is held at each level, as indicated by the points, for a few seconds to allow the lung to come to rest. In this way, the pressure-volume curve of the lung can be plotted.

In Figure 7.3, the expanding pressure around the lung is generated by a pump, but in man it is developed by an increase in volume of the chest cage. The fact that the intrapleural space between the lung and

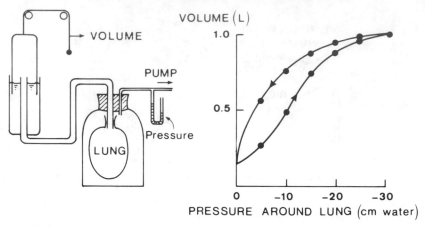

Figure 7.3. Measurement of the pressure-volume curve of excised lung. The lung is held at each pressure for a few seconds while its volume is measured. The curve is nonlinear and becomes flatter at high expanding pressures. Note that the inflation and deflation curves are not the same; this is called hysteresis.

chest wall is much smaller than the space between the lung and the bottle in Figure 7.3 makes no essential difference. The intrapleural space contains only a few milliliters of fluid.

Figure 7.3 shows that the curves which the lung follows during inflation and deflation are different. This behavior is known as *hysteresis.* Note that the lung volume at any given pressure during deflation is larger than during inflation. Note also that the lung without any expanding pressure has some air inside it. In fact even if the pressure around the lung is raised above atmospheric pressure, little further air is lost because small airways close, trapping gas in the alveoli (compare Figure 7.9). This *airway closure* occurs at higher lung volumes with increasing age and also in some types of lung disease.

In Figure 7.3 the pressure inside the airways and alveoli of the lung is the same as atmospheric pressure, which is zero on the X axis. Thus, this axis also measures the difference in pressure between the inside and outside of the lung. This is known as *transpulmonary pressure* and is numerically equal to the pressure around the lung when the alveolar pressure is atmospheric. It is also possible to measure the pressure-volume of the lung shown in Figure 7.3 by inflating it with positive pressure and leaving the pleural surface exposed to the atmosphere. In this case, the X axis could be labeled "airway pressure," and the values would be positive. The curves would be identical to those shown in Figure 7.3.

Compliance

The slope of the pressure-volume curve, or the volume change per unit pressure change is known as the *compliance*. In the normal range (expanding pressure of about -2 to -10 cm water) the lung is remarkably distensible or very compliant. The compliance of the human lung is about 200 ml/cm water. However, at high expanding pressures, the lung is stiffer, and its compliance is smaller, as shown by the flatter slope of the curve.

The compliance is *reduced* somewhat if the pulmonary venous pressure is increased and the lung becomes engorged with blood. Alveolar edema decreases compliance by preventing the inflation of some alveoli. The compliance also apparently falls if the lung remains unventilated for a long period, especially if its volume is low. This may be partly caused by atelectasis of some lung units, but increases in surface tension also occur (see below). Diseases causing fibrosis of the lung decrease compliance. The compliance of the lung is *increased* by age and also by emphysema. In both instances, an alteration in the elastic tissue of the lung is probably responsible.

The compliance of lung depends on its size. Clearly, the change in volume per unit change of pressure will be larger for a human lung than, say, a mouse lung. For this reason, the compliance per unit volume of lung, or *specific compliance*, is sometimes measured if we wish to draw conclusions about the elastic properties of the lung tissue.

The pressure surrounding the lung is less than atmospheric in Figure 7.3 (and in the living chest) because of the elastic recoil of the lung. What is responsible for the lung's elastic behavior, that is, its tendency to return to its resting volume after distension? One factor is the elastic tissue which is visible in histological sections. Fibers of elastin and collagen can be seen in the alveolar walls and around vessels and bronchi. Probably the elastic behavior of the lung has less to do with simple elongation of these fibers than with their geometrical arrangement. An analogy is a nylon stocking which is very distensible because of its knitted make-up, although the individual nylon fibers are very difficult to stretch. The changes in elastic recoil that occur in the lung with age and in emphysema are presumably caused by changes in this elastic tissue.

Surface Tension

Another very important factor in the pressure-volume behavior of lung is the surface tension of the liquid film lining the alveoli.

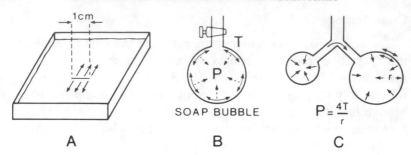

Figure 7.4. (A) Surface tension is the force (in dynes, for example) acting across an imaginary line 1 cm long in a liquid surface. (B) Surface forces in a soap bubble tend to reduce the area of the surface and generate a pressure within the bubble. (C) Because the smaller bubble generates a larger pressure, it blows up the large bubble.

Surface tension is the force (in dynes, for example) acting across an imaginary line 1 cm long in the surface of the liquid (Figure 7.4A). It arises because the forces between adjacent molecules of the liquid are much stronger than those between the liquid and gas, with the result that the liquid surface area becomes as small as possible. This behavior is seen clearly in a soap bubble blown on the end of a tube (Figure 7.4B). The surfaces of the bubble contract as much as they can, forming a sphere (smallest surface area for a given volume) and generating a pressure which can be predicted from Laplace's law: pressure = (4 × surface tension)/radius. When only one surface is involved in a liquid-lined spherical alveolus, the numerator has the number 2 rather than 4.

The first evidence that surface tension might contribute to the pressure-volume behavior of the lung was obtained by von Neergaard when he showed that lungs inflated with saline have a much larger compliance (are easier to distend) than air-filled lungs (Figure 7.5). Since the saline abolished the surface tension forces but presumably did not affect the tissue forces of the lung, this observation meant that surface tension contributed a large part of the static recoil force of the lung. Some time later, workers studying edema foam coming from the lungs of animals exposed to noxious gases noticed that the tiny air bubbles of the foam were extremely stable. They recognized that this indicated a very low surface tension, an observation which led to the remarkable discovery of pulmonary *surfactant*.

It is now known that some of the cells lining the alveoli secrete a material which profoundly lowers the surface tension of the alveolar lining fluid. The exact nature of this material is not known, but

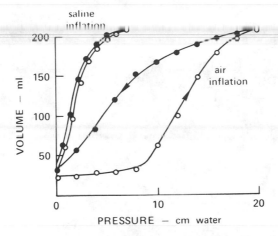

Figure 7.5. Comparison of pressure-volume curves of air-filled and saline-filled lungs (cat). *Open circles,* inflation; *closed circles,* deflation. Note that the saline-filled lung has a higher compliance and also much less hysteresis than the air-filled lung. (From EP Radford: *Tissue Elasticity.* Washington, DC, American Physiological Society, 1957, p 177.)

dipalmitoyl phosphatidyl choline (DPPC) is an important constituent. Alveolar epithelial cells are of two types. Type I cells have the shape of a fried egg with long cytoplasmic extensions spreading out thinly over the alveolar walls (Figure 1.1). Type II cells are more compact (Figure 7.6), and electron microscopy shows osmiophilic lamellated bodies within them which are extruded into the alveoli and transform into surfactant. Some of the surfactant can be washed out of animal lungs by rinsing them with saline.

The phospholipid DPPC is synthesized in the lung from fatty acids which are either extracted from the blood or are themselves synthesized in the lung. Synthesis is fast, and there is a rapid turnover of surfactant. If the blood flow to a region of lung is abolished as the result of an embolus, for example, the surfactant there may be depleted. Surfactant is formed relatively late in fetal life, and babies born without adequate amounts develop respiratory distress and may die.

The effects of this material on surface tension can be studied with a surface balance (Figure 7.7). This consists of a tray containing saline on which a small amount of test material is placed. The area of the surface is then alternately expanded and compressed by a movable barrier while the surface tension is measured from the force exerted on a platinum strip. Pure saline gives a surface tension of

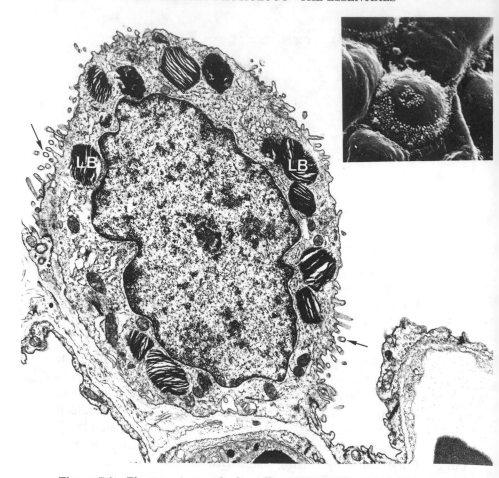

Figure 7.6.   Electron micrograph of type II epithelial cell (× 10,000). Note the osmiophilic lamellated bodies (*LB*), large nucleus, and microvilli (*arrows*). The *inset* at *top right* is a scanning electron micrograph showing the surface view of a type II cell with its characteristic distribution of microvilli (× 3400). (From ER Weibel and J Gil: In JB West: *Bioengineering Aspects of the Lung*. New York, Marcel Dekker, 1977, p 15.)

about 70 dynes/cm, irrespective of the area of its surface. Adding detergent reduces the surface tension, but again this is independent of area. When lung washings are placed on saline, the curve shown in Figure 7.7*B* is obtained. Note that the surface tension changes greatly with the surface area and that there is hysteresis (compare Figure 7.3). Note also that the surface tension falls to extremely low values when the area is small.

How does surfactant reduce the surface tension so much? Appar-

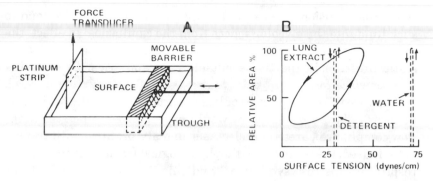

Figure 7.7. (A) Surface balance. The area of the surface is altered, and the surface tension is measured from the force exerted on a platinum strip dipped into the surface. (B) Plots of surface tension and area obtained with a surface balance. Note that lung washings show a change in surface tension with area and that the minimum tension is very small.

ently the molecules of DPPC are hydrophobic at one end and hydrophilic at the other, and they align themselves in the surface. When this occurs, their intermolecular repulsive forces oppose the normal attracting forces between surface molecules which are responsible for surface tension. The reduction in surface tension is greater when the film is compressed because the molecules of DPPC are then crowded closer together and repel each other more.

What are the physiological advantages of surfactant? First, a low surface tension in the alveoli increases the compliance of the lung and reduces the work of expanding it with each breath. Next, stability of the alveoli is promoted. The 300 million alveoli appear to be inherently unstable because areas of atelectasis (collapse) often form in the presence of disease. This is a complex subject, but one way of looking at the lung is to regard it as a collection of millions of tiny bubbles (although this is clearly an oversimplification). In such an arrangement, there is a tendency for small bubbles to collapse and blow up large ones. Figure 7.4C shows that the pressure generated by the surface forces in a bubble is inversely proportional to its radius, with the result that if the surface tensions are the same, the pressure inside a small bubble exceeds that in a large bubble. However, Figure 7.7 shows that when lung washings are present, a small surface area is associated with a small surface tension. Thus, the tendency for small alveoli to empty into large alveoli is apparently reduced.

A third role of surfactant is to help to keep the alveoli dry. Just as the surface tension forces tend to collapse alveoli, they also tend to suck fluid into the alveolar spaces from the capillaries. In effect, the surface tension of the curved alveolar surface reduces the hydrostatic pressure in the tissue outside the capillaries. By reducing these surface forces, surfactant prevents the transudation of fluid.

What are the consequences of loss of surfactant? On the basis of its functions discussed above, we would expect these to be stiff lungs (low compliance), areas of atelectasis, and alveoli filled with transudate. Indeed, these are the pathophysiological features of the "infant respiratory distress syndrome," and this disease is thought to be caused by an absence of this crucial material.

There is another mechanism that apparently contributes to the stability of the alveoli in the lung. Figures 1.2, 1.7, and 4.3 remind us that all the alveoli (except those immediately adjacent to the pleural surface) are surrounded by other alveoli and are therefore supported by each other. In a structure such as this with many connecting links, any tendency for one group of units to reduce or increase its volume relative to the rest of the structure is opposed. For example, if a group of alveoli has a tendency to collapse, large expanding forces will be developed on them by virtue of the fact that the surrounding parenchyma is expanded.

This support offered to lung units by those surrounding them is termed "interdependence." The same factors explain the development of low pressures around large blood vessels and airways as the lung expands (Figure 4.2). Some physiologists believe that the role of interdependence may be more important than that of surfactant in maintaining the stability of the small air spaces.

CAUSE OF REGIONAL DIFFERENCES IN VENTILATION

We saw in Figure 2.7 that the lower regions of the lung ventilate more than the upper zones, and this is a convenient place to discuss the cause of these topographical differences. It has been shown that the intrapleural pressure is less negative at the bottom than the top of the lung (Figure 7.8). The probable reason for this is the weight of the lung. Anything that is supported requires a larger pressure below it than above it to balance the downward-acting weight forces, and the lung, which is partly supported by the rib cage and diaphragm, is no exception. Thus the pressure near the base is higher (less negative) than at the apex.

Figure 7.8 shows the way in which the volume of a portion of lung (for example, a lobe) expands as the pressure around it is decreased (compare Figure 7.1). The pressure inside the lung is the same as atmospheric pressure. Note that the lung is easier to inflate at low volumes than at high volumes, where it becomes stiffer. Because the expanding pressure at the base of the lung is small, this region has a small resting volume. However, because it is situated on a steep part of the pressure-volume curve, it expands well on inspiration. By contrast, the apex of the lung has a large expanding pressure, a big resting volume, and small change in volume on inspiration.*

Now when we talk of regional differences in ventilation, we mean the change in volume per unit resting volume. It is clear from Figure 7.8 that the base of the lung has both a larger change in volume and smaller resting volume than the apex. Thus, its ventilation is greater. Note the paradox that although the base of the lung is relatively poorly expanded compared with the apex, it is better ventilated. The same explanation can be given for the large ventilation of dependent lung in both the supine and lateral positions.

A remarkable change in the distribution of ventilation occurs at low lung volumes. Figure 7.9 is similar to Figure 7.8 except that it represents the situation at residual volume (that is, after a full expiration, Figure 2.2). Now the intrapleural pressures are less negative because the lung is not so well expanded and the elastic recoil forces are smaller. However, the differences between apex and base are still present because of the weight of the lung. Note that the intrapleural pressure at the base now actually exceeds airway (atmospheric) pressure. Under these conditions the lung at the base is not being expanded but compressed, and ventilation is impossible until the local intrapleural pressure falls below atmospheric pressure. By contrast the apex of the lung is on a favorable part of the pressure-volume curve and ventilates well. Thus the normal distribution of ventilation is inverted, the upper regions ventilating better than the lower zones.

Airway Closure

The compressed region of lung at the base does not have all its gas squeezed out. In practice, small airways, probably in the region of respiratory bronchioles (Figure 1.4), close first, thus trapping gas in the distal alveoli. This *airway closure* only occurs at very low lung

---

* This explanation is an oversimplification because the pressure-volume behavior of a portion of a structure like the lung may not be identical to that of the whole organ.

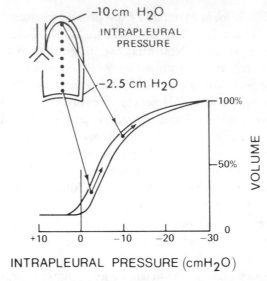

Figure 7.8. An explanation of the regional differences of ventilation down the lung. Because of the weight of the lung, the intrapleural pressure is less negative at the base than at the apex. As a consequence, the basal lung is relatively compressed in its resting state but expands better on inspiration than the apex. (From JB West: *Ventilation/Blood Flow and Gas Exchange,* ed 4. Oxford, Blackwell, 1985.)

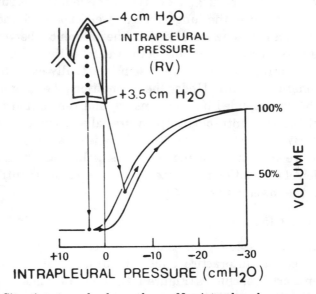

Figure 7.9. Situation at very low lung volumes. Now intrapleural pressures are less negative, and the pressure at the base actually exceeds airway (atmospheric) pressure. As a consequence airway closure occurs in this region, and no gas enters with small inspirations. (From JB West: *Ventilation/Blood Flow and Gas Exchange,* ed 4. Oxford, Blackwell, 1985.)

volumes in young normal subjects. However, in elderly apparently normal people, airway closure in the lowermost regions of the lung occurs at higher volumes and may be present at functional residual capacity (Figure 2.2). The reason for this is that the aging lung loses some of its elastic recoil, and intrapleural pressures therefore become less negative, thus approaching the situation shown in Figure 7.9. In these circumstances, dependent regions of the lung may be only intermittently ventilated, and this leads to defective gas exchange (Chapter 5). A similar situation frequently develops in patients with some types of chronic lung disease.

ELASTIC PROPERTIES OF THE CHEST WALL

Just as the lung is elastic, so is the thoracic cage. This can be illustrated by putting air into the intrapleural space (pneumothorax). Figure 7.10 shows that the normal pressure outside the lung is subatmospheric just as it is in the jar of Figure 7.3. When air is introduced into the intrapleural space, raising the pressure to atmospheric, the lung collapses inward, and the chest wall springs outward. This shows that under equilibrium conditions, the chest wall is pulled inward while the lung is pulled outward, the two pulls balancing each other.

These interactions can be seen more clearly if we plot a pressure-volume curve for the lung and chest wall (Figure 7.11). For this, the subject inspires or expires from a spirometer and then relaxes his respiratory muscles while the airway pressure is measured ("relaxation pressure"). Incidentally, this is difficult for an untrained subject. Figure 7.11 shows that at functional residual capacity (FRC), the relaxation pressure of the lung and chest wall is atmospheric. Indeed FRC is the equilibrium volume when the elastic recoil of the lung is balanced by the normal tendency for the chest wall to spring

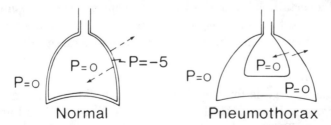

Figure 7.10. The tendency of the lung to recoil to its deflated volume is balanced by the tendency of the chest cage to bow out. As a result, the intrapleural pressure is subatmospheric. Pneumothorax allows the lung to collapse and the thorax to spring out.

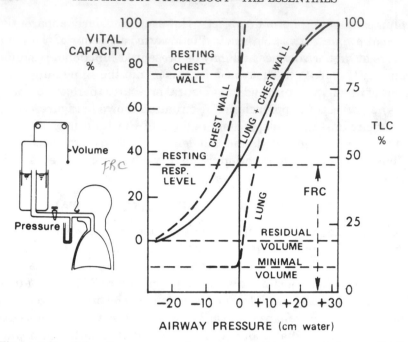

Figure 7.11. Relaxation pressure-volume curve of the lung and chest wall. The subject inspires (or expires) to a certain volume from the spirometer, the tap is closed, and he then relaxes his respiratory muscles. The curve for lung + chest wall can be explained by the addition of the individual lung and chest wall curves. (Modified from H Rahn et al: *Am J Physiol* 146:161, 1946.)

out. At volumes above this, the pressure is positive, and at smaller volumes, the pressure is subatmospheric. Also shown is the curve for the lung alone. This is similar to that shown in Figure 7.3, except that for clarity no hysteresis is indicated and the pressure are positive instead of negative. They are the pressures which would be found from the experiment of Figure 7.3 if, after the lung had reached a certain volume, the line to the spirometer were clamped, the jar opened to the atmosphere (so that the lung relaxed against the closed airway), and the airway pressure measured. Note that at zero pressure the lung is at its minimal volume, which is below residual volume (RV).

The third curve is for the chest wall only. We can imagine this being measured on a subject with a normal chest wall and no lung! Note that at FRC the relaxation pressure is negative. In other words, at this volume the chest cage is tending to spring out. It is not until the volume is increased to about 75% of the vital capacity that the relaxation pressure is atmospheric, that is, that the chest wall has found its equilibrium position. At every volume, the relaxation pressure of the lung plus chest wall is the sum of the pressures for the lung and the chest wall measured separately. Since the pressure (at a given volume) is inversely proportional to compliance, this implies that the total compliance of the lung and chest wall is the sum of the reciprocals of the lung and chest wall compliances measured separately, or $1/C_T = 1/C_L + 1/C_{CW}$.

AIRWAY RESISTANCE

Airflow through Tubes

If air flows through a tube (Figure 7.12), a difference of pressure exists between the ends. The pressure difference depends on the rate and pattern of flow. At low flow rates, the stream lines may everywhere be parallel to the sides of the tube (A). This is known as laminar flow. As the flow rate is increased, unsteadiness develops, especially at branches. Here, separation of the stream lines from the wall may occur with the formation of local eddies (B). At still higher flow rates, complete disorganization of the stream lines is seen; this is turbulence (C).

The pressure-flow characteristics for *laminar flow* were first described by the French physician Poiseuille. In straight circular tubes, the volume flow rate is given by

$$\dot{V} = \frac{P\pi r^4}{8nl}$$

where P is the driving pressure (ΔP in Figure 7.12A), r radius, n viscosity, and l length. It can be seen that driving pressure is proportional to flow rate, or $P = K\dot{V}$. Since flow resistance R is driving pressure divided by flow (compare p. 35), we have

$$R = \frac{8nl}{\pi r^4}$$

Note the critical importance of tube radius; if the radius is halved, the resistance increases 16-fold! However, doubling the length only doubles resistance. Note also that the viscosity of the gas, but not its density, affects the pressure-flow relationship.

Another feature of laminar flow when it is fully developed is that the gas in the center of the tube moves twice as fast as the average velocity. Thus, a spike of rapidly moving gas travels down the axis of the tube (Figure 7.12A). This changing velocity across the diameter of the tube is known as the *velocity profile*.

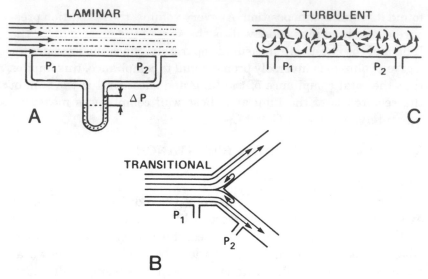

Figure 7.12.   Patterns of airflow in tubes. In A the flow is laminar, in B transitional with eddy formation at branches, and in C turbulent. Resistance is $(P_1 - P_2)$/flow.

Turbulent flow has different properties. Here pressure is not proportional to flow rate but, approximately, to its square: $P = K\dot{V}^2$. In addition, the viscosity of the gas becomes relatively unimportant, but an increase in gas density increases the pressure drop for a given flow. Turbulent flow does not have the high axial flow velocity that is characteristic of laminar flow.

Whether flow will be laminar or turbulent depends to a large extent on the Reynolds number, Re. This is given by

$$Re = \frac{2rvd}{n}$$

where d is density, v average velocity, r radius, and n viscosity. In straight smooth tubes, turbulence is probable when the Reynolds number exceeds 2000. The expression shows that turbulence is most likely to occur when the velocity of flow is high and the tube diameter is large (for a given velocity). Note also that a low-density gas like helium tends to produce less turbulence.

In such a complicated system of tubes as the bronchial tree with its many branches, changes in caliber, and irregular wall surfaces, the application of the above principles is difficult. In practice, for laminar flow to occur the entrance conditions of the tube are critical. If eddy formation occurs upstream at a branch point, this disturbance is carried downstream some distance before it disappears. Thus in a rapidly branching system like the lung, fully developed laminar flow (Figure 7.12A) probably only occurs in the very small airways where the Reynolds numbers are very low (approximately 1 in terminal bronchioles). In most of the bronchial tree, flow is transitional (B), while true turbulence may occur in the trachea, especially on exercise when flow velocities are high. In general, driving pressure is determined by both the flow rate and its square: $P = K_1\dot{V} + K_2\dot{V}^2$.

Measurement of Airway Resistance

Airway resistance is the pressure difference between the alveoli and the mouth divided by flow rate (Figure 7.12). Mouth pressure is easily measured with a manometer. Alveolar pressure can be deduced from measurements made in a body plethysmograph. Details of this technique are given on p. 158.

Pressures during the Breathing Cycle

Suppose we measure the pressures in the intrapleural and alveolar spaces during normal breathing.† Figure 7.13 shows that before inspiration begins, the intrapleural pressure is −5 cm water because of the elastic recoil of the lung (compare Figures 7.3 and 7.10). Alveolar pressure is zero (atmospheric) because with no airflow, there is no pressure drop along the airways. However, for inspiratory flow to occur, the alveolar pressure falls, thus establishing the driving pressure (Figure 7.12). Indeed, the extent of the fall depends on the flow rate and the resistance of the airways. In normal subjects, the change in alveolar pressure is only 1 cm water or so, but in patients with airway obstruction, it may be many times that.

Intrapleural pressure falls during inspiration for two reasons. First, as the lung expands, its elastic recoil increases (Figure 7.3). This alone would cause the intrapleural pressure to move along the broken line ABC. In addition, however, the pressure drop along the airway is associated with a further fall in intrapleural pressure,‡ represented by the hatched area, so that the actual path is AB′C. Thus, the vertical distance between lines ABC and AB′C reflects the alveolar pressure at any instant. As an equation of pressures

---

† Intrapleural pressure can be measured by placing a balloon catheter in the esophagus.

‡ There is also a small contribution made by tissue resistance which is considered later in this chapter.

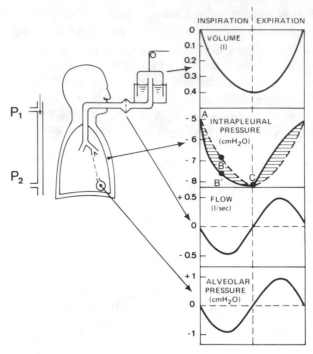

Figure 7.13. Pressures during the breathing cycle. If there were no airway resistance, alveolar pressure would remain at zero, and intrapleural pressure would follow the *broken line ABC*, which is determined by the elastic recoil of the lung. Airway (and tissue) resistance contributes the *hatched portion* of intrapleural pressure (see text).

(mouth-intrapleural) = (mouth-alveolar) + (alveolar-intrapleural).

On expiration, similar changes occur. Now intrapleural pressure is *less* negative than it would be in the absence of airway resistance because alveolar pressure is positive. Indeed, with a forced expiration intrapleural pressure goes above zero.

Note that the shape of the alveolar pressure tracing is similar to that of flow. Indeed, they would be identical if the airway resistance remained constant during the cycle. Also the intrapleural pressure curve ABC would have the same shape as the volume tracing if the lung compliance remained constant.

Chief Site of Airway Resistance

As the airways penetrate toward the periphery of the lung, they become more numerous but much narrower (see Figures 1.3–1.5).

Based on Poiseuille's equation with its (radius)^4 term, it would be natural to think that the major part of the resistance lies in the very narrow airways. Indeed, this was thought to be the case for many years. However, it has now been shown by direct measurements of the pressure drop along the bronchial tree that the major site of resistance is the medium-sized bronchi and that the very small bronchioles contribute relatively little resistance. Figure 7.14 shows that most of the pressure drop occurs in the airways up to the seventh generation. Less than 20% can be attributed to airways less than 2 mm in diameter. The reason for this apparent paradox is the prodigious number of small airways.

The fact that the peripheral airways contribute so little resistance is important in the detection of early airway disease. Because they constitute a "silent zone" it is probable that considerable small airway disease can be present before the usual measurements of airway resistance can pick up an abnormality. This question is considered in more detail in Chapter 10.

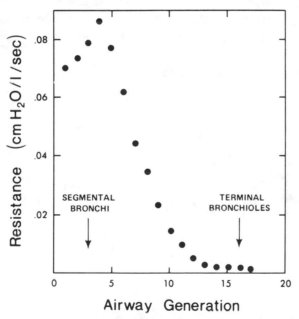

Figure 7.14. Location of the chief site of airway resistance. Note that the intermediate-sized bronchi contribute most of the resistance and that relatively little is located in the very small airways. (Redrawn from TJ Pedley et al: *Respir Physiol* 9:387, 1970.)

Factors Determining Airway Resistance

Lung volume has an important effect on airway resistance. Like the extra-alveolar blood vessels (Figure 4.2), the bronchi are supported by the radial traction of the surrounding lung tissue, and their caliber is increased as the lung expands (compare Figure 4.6). Figure 7.15 shows that as lung volume is reduced, airway resistance rises rapidly. If the reciprocal of resistance (conductance) is plotted against lung volume, an approximately linear relationship is obtained.

At very low lung volumes, the small airways may close completely, especially at the bottom of the lung, where the lung is less well expanded (Figure 7.9). Patients who have increased airway resistance often breathe at high lung volumes; this helps to reduce their airway resistance.

Contraction of *bronchial smooth muscle* narrows the airways and increases airway resistance. This may occur reflexly through the stimulation of receptors in the trachea and large bronchi by irritants such as cigarette smoke. Motor innervation is by the vagus nerve. The tone of the smooth muscle is under the control of the autonomic nervous system. Sympathetic stimulation causes bronchodilatation as do the drugs isoproterenol, epinephrine, and norepinephrine.

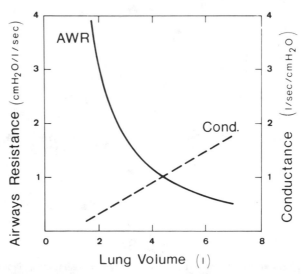

Figure 7.15. Variation of airway resistance with lung volume. If the reciprocal of airway resistance (conductance) is plotted, the graph is a straight line. (Redrawn from WA Briscoe and AB Dubois: *J Clin Invest* 37:1279, 1958.)

Parasympathetic activity causes bronchoconstriction, as does acetyl-choline. A fall of P_{CO_2} in alveolar gas causes an increase in airway resistance, apparently as a result of a direct action on bronchiolar smooth muscle. The injection of histamine into the pulmonary artery causes constriction of smooth muscle located in the alveolar ducts.

The *density* and *viscosity* of the inspired gas affect the resistance offered to flow. The resistance is increased during a deep dive because the increased pressure raises gas density, but it is reduced when a helium-O_2 mixture is breathed. The fact that changes in density rather than viscosity have such an influence on resistance is evidence that flow is not purely laminar in the medium-sized airways, where the main site of resistance lies (Figure 7.14).

Dynamic Compression of Airways

Suppose a subject inspires to total lung capacity and then exhales as hard as he can to residual volume. We can record a *flow-volume curve* like A in Figure 7.16 which shows that flow rises very rapidly to a high value but then declines over most of expiration. A remarkable feature of this flow-volume envelope is that it is virtually impossible to penetrate it. For example, no matter whether we start exhaling slowly and then accelerate, as in B, or make a less forceful expiration, as in C, the descending portion of the flow-volume curve

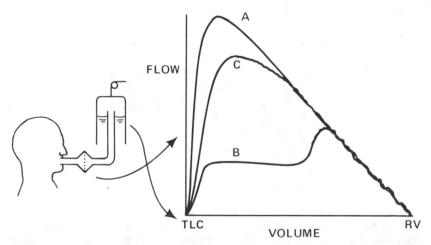

Figure 7.16. Flow-volume curves. In *A*, a maximal inspiration was followed by a forced expiration. In *B*, expiration was initially slow and then forced. In *C*, expiratory effort was submaximal. In all three, the descending portions of the curves are almost superimposed.

takes virtually the same path. Thus, something powerful is limiting expiratory flow, and over most of the lung volume, flow rate is independent of effort.

   We can get more information about this curious state of affairs by plotting the data in another way, as shown in Figure 7.17. For this the subject takes a series of maximal inspirations (or expirations), and then exhales (or inhales) fully with varying degrees of effort. If the flow rates and intrapleural pressures are plotted at the *same* lung volume for each expiration and inspiration, so-called *isovolume pressure-flow curves* can be obtained. It can be seen that at high lung volumes, the expiratory flow rate continues to increase with effort as might be expected. However, at mid or low volumes, the flow rate reaches a plateau and cannot be increased with further increase in intrapleural pressure. Under these conditions, flow is therefore *effort independent*.

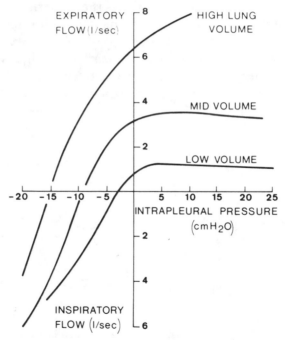

Figure 7.17. Isovolume pressure-flow curves drawn for three lung volumes. Each of these was obtained from a series of forced expirations and inspirations (see text). Note that at the high lung volume, a rise in intrapleural pressure (obtained by increasing expiratory effort) results in a greater expiratory flow. However, at mid and low volumes, flow becomes independent of effort after a certain intrapleural pressure has been exceeded. (Redrawn from DL Fry and RE Hyatt: *Am J Med* 29:672, 1960.)

The reason for this remarkable behavior is compression of the airways by intrathoracic pressure. Figure 7.18 shows schematically the forces acting across an airway within the lung. The pressure outside the airway is shown as intrapleural, although this is an oversimplification. In *A*, before inspiration has begun, airway pressure is everywhere zero (no flow), and since intrapleural pressure is −5 cm water, there is a pressure of 5 cm water holding the airway open. As inspiration starts (*B*), both intrapleural and alveolar pressure fall by 2 cm water (same lung volume as *A* and tissue resistance is neglected), and flow begins. Because of the pressure drop along the airway, the pressure inside is −1 cm water, and there is a pressure of 6 cm water holding the airway open. At end-inspiration (*C*), again flow is zero, and there is an airway transmural pressure of 8 cm water.

Finally, at the onset of forced expiration (*D*), both intrapleural pressure and alveolar pressure increase by 38 cm water (same lung volume as *C*). Because of the pressure drop along the airway as flow begins, there is now a pressure of 11 cm water tending to *close* the airway. Airway collapse occurs, and the downstream pressure limiting flow becomes the pressure outside the airway, or intrapleural pressure. Thus, the effective driving pressure becomes alveolar minus intrapleural pressure. This is the same Starling resistor

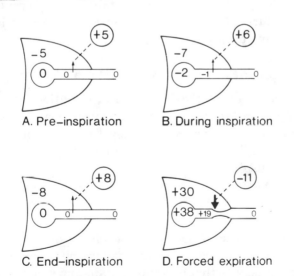

Figure 7.18. Scheme showing why airways are compressed during forced expiration. Note that the pressure difference across the airway is holding it open, except during a forced expiration. See text for details.

mechanism which limits the blood flow in zone 2 of the lung, where venous pressure becomes unimportant just as mouth pressure does here (Figures 4.9 and 4.10). Note that if intrapleural pressure is raised further by increased muscular effort in an attempt to expel gas, the effective driving pressure is unaltered. Thus flow is independent of effort.

Maximum flow decreases with lung volume (Figure 7.16) because the difference between alveolar and intrapleural pressure decreases and also the airways become narrower. Note also that flow is independent of the resistance of the airways downstream of the point of collapse, sometimes called the *equal pressure point.* As expiration progresses the equal pressure point moves distally, deeper into the lung. This occurs because the resistance of the airways rises as lung volume falls, and therefore the pressure within the airways falls more rapidly with distance from the alveoli.

Several factors exaggerate this flow-limiting mechanism. One is any increase in resistance of the peripheral airways since that magnifies the pressure drop along them and thus decreases the intrabronchial pressure during expiration (19 cm water in *D*). Another is a low lung volume because that reduces the driving pressure (alveolar-intrapleural). This driving pressure is also reduced if compliance is increased, as in emphysema. Indeed, while this type of flow limitation is only seen during forced expiration in normal subjects, it may occur during the expirations of normal breathing in patients with severe lung disease.

CAUSES OF UNEVEN VENTILATION

The cause of the regional differences in ventilation in the lung was discussed on p. 96. Apart from these topographical differences it is probable that at any given vertical level there is some additional inequality of ventilation in the normal lung, and this is certainly the case in many diseases.

One mechanism of uneven ventilation is shown in Figure 7.19. If we regard a lung unit (Figure 2.1) as an elastic chamber connected to the atmosphere by a tube, the amount of ventilation depends on the compliance of the chamber and the resistance of the tube. In Figure 7.19, unit *A* has a normal distensibility and airway resistance. It can be seen that its volume change on inspiration is large and rapid so that it is complete before expiration for the whole lung

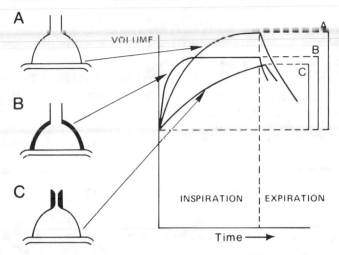

Figure 7.19. Effects of decreased compliance (*B*) and increased airway resistance (*C*) on ventilation of lung units compared with normal (*A*). In both instances the inspired volume is abnormally low. (Modified from JB West: *Ventilation/Blood Flow and Gas Exchange,* ed 4. Oxford, Blackwell, 1985.)

begins (*broken line*). By contrast unit *B* has a low compliance, and its change in volume is rapid but small. Finally, unit *C* has a large airway resistance so that inspiration is slow and not complete before the lung has begun to exhale. Note that the shorter the time available for inspiration (fast breathing rate), the smaller the inspired volume. Such a unit is said to have a long *time constant,* the value of which is given by the product of the compliance and resistance. Thus, inequality of ventilation can result either from alterations in local distensibility or airway resistance, and the pattern of inequality will depend on the frequency of breathing.

Another possible mechanism of uneven ventilation is incomplete diffusion within the airways of the respiratory zone (Figure 1.4). We saw in Chapter 1 that the dominant mechanism of ventilation of the lung beyond the terminal bronchioles is diffusion. Normally this occurs so rapidly that differences in gas concentration in the acinus are virtually abolished within a fraction of a second. However, if there is dilatation of the airways in the region of the respiratory bronchioles, as in some diseases, the distance to be covered by diffusion may be enormously increased. In these circumstances, inspired gas is not distributed uniformly within the respiratory zone because of uneven ventilation *along* the lung units.

TISSUE RESISTANCE

When the lung and chest wall are moved, some pressure is required to overcome the viscous forces within the tissues as they slide over each other. Thus, part of the hatched portion of Figure 7.13 should be attributed to these tissue forces. However, this tissue resistance is only about 20% of the total (tissue + airway) resistance in young normal subjects, although it may increase in some diseases. This total resistance is sometimes called *pulmonary resistance* to distinguish it from airway resistance.

WORK OF BREATHING

Work is required to move the lung and chest wall. In this context, it is most convenient to measure work as pressure × volume.

Work Done on the Lung

This can be illustrated on a pressure-volume curve (Figure 7.20). During inspiration, the intrapleural pressure follows the curve ABC, and the work done on the lung is given by the area 0ABCD0. Of this, the trapezoid 0AECD0 represents the work required to overcome the elastic forces, and the hatched area ABCEA represents the work overcoming viscous (airway and tissue) resistance (compare Figure 7.13). The higher the airway resistance or the inspiratory flow rate, the more negative (rightward) would be the intrapleural pressure excursion between A and C and the larger the area.

On expiration, the area AECFA is the work required to overcome airway (+tissue) resistance. Normally, this falls within the trape-

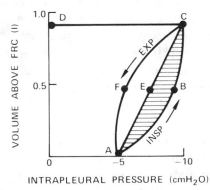

Figure 7.20. Pressure-volume curve of the lung showing the inspiratory work done overcoming elastic forces (*area 0AECD0*) and viscous forces (*hatched area ABCEA*).

zoid 0AECD0, and thus this work can be accomplished by the energy stored in the expanded elastic structures and released during a passive expiration. The difference between the areas AECFA and 0AECD0 represents the work dissipated as heat.

The higher the breathing rate, the faster the flow rates and the larger the viscous work area ABCEA. On the other hand, the larger the tidal volume, the larger the elastic work area (0AECD0. It is of interest that patients who have a reduced compliance (stiff lungs) tend to take small rapid breaths, while patients with severe airway obstruction often breathe slowly. These patterns tend to reduce the work done on the lungs.

Total Work of Breathing

The total work done moving the lung and chest wall is difficult to measure, although estimates have been obtained by artifically ventilating paralyzed patients (or "completely relaxed" volunteers) in an iron lung type of respirator. Alternatively, the total work can be calculated by measuring the O_2 cost of breathing and assuming a figure for the *efficiency* as given by:

$$\text{Efficiency } \% = \frac{\text{Useful work}}{\text{Total energy expended (or } O_2 \text{ cost)}} \times 100$$

The efficiency is believed to be about 5–10%.

The O_2 cost of quiet breathing is extremely small, being less than 5% of the total resting O_2 consumption. With voluntary hyperventilation it is possible to increase this to 30%. In patients with obstructive lung disease, the O_2 cost of breathing may limit their exercise ability.

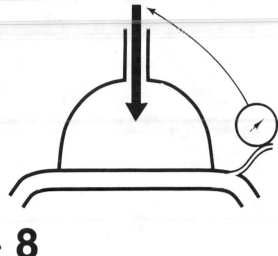

chapter 8

Control of Ventilation

how gas exchange is regulated

We have seen that the chief function of the lung is to exchange O_2 and CO_2 between blood and gas and thus maintain normal levels of P_{O_2} and P_{CO_2} in arterial blood. In this chapter we shall see that in spite of widely differing demands for O_2 uptake and CO_2 output made by the body, the arterial P_{O_2} and P_{CO_2} are normally kept within close limits. This remarkable regulation of gas exchange is possible because the level of ventilation is so carefully controlled.

The three basic elements of the respiratory control system (Figure 8.1) are:

1. *Sensors* which gather information and feed it to the
2. *Central controller* in the brain which coordinates the information and, in turn, sends impulses to the
3. *Effectors* (respiratory muscles) which cause ventilation.

We shall see that increased activity of the effectors generally ulti-

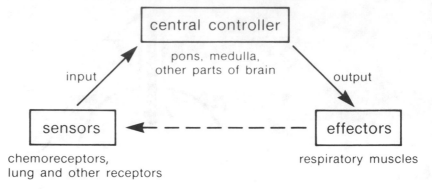

Figure 8.1. Basic elements of the respiratory control system. Information from various sensors is fed to the central controller, the output of which goes to the respiratory muscles. By changing ventilation, the respiratory muscles reduce perturbations of the sensors (negative feedback).

mately decreases the sensory input to the brain, for example, by decreasing the arterial P_{CO_2}. This is an example of negative feedback.

CENTRAL CONTROLLER

The normal automatic process of breathing originates in impulses that come from the brainstem. The cortex can override these centers if voluntary control is desired. Additional input from other parts of the brain occurs under certain conditions.

Brainstem

The periodic nature of inspiration and expiration is controlled by neurons located in the pons and medulla. These have been designated the *respiratory centers*. However, these should not be thought of as comprising a discrete nucleus but rather as a somewhat poorly defined collection of neurons with various components.

Three main groups of neurons are recognized.

1. *Medullary respiratory* center in the reticular formation of the medulla. This is comprised of two identifiable areas. One group of cells in the dorsal region of the medulla (dorsal respiratory group) is chiefly associated with inspiration; the other in the ventral area (ventral respiratory group) is mainly for expiration. One popular (though not universally accepted) view is that the cells of the *inspiratory area* have the property of intrinsic periodic firing, and they are responsible for the basic rhythm of ventilation. When all known afferent stimuli have been abolished, these inspiratory cells gener-

ate repetitive bursts of action potentials that result in nervous impulses going to the diaphragm and other inspiratory muscles.

The intrinsic rhythm pattern of the inspiratory area starts with a latent period of several seconds during which there is no activity. Action potentials then begin to appear, increasing in a crescendo over the next few seconds. During this time, inspiratory muscle activity becomes stronger in a "ramp"-type pattern. Finally, the inspiratory action potentials cease, and inspiratory muscle tone falls to its preinspiratory level.

The inspiratory ramp can be "turned off" prematurely by inhibiting impulses from the *pneumotaxic center* (see below). In this way inspiration is shortened and, as a consequence, the breathing rate increases. The output of the inspiratory cells is further modulated by impulses from the vagal and glossopharyngeal nerves. Indeed, these terminate in the tractus solitarius, which is situated close to the inspiratory area.

The *expiratory area* is quiescent during normal quiet breathing because ventilation is then achieved by active contraction of the inspiratory muscles (chiefly the diaphragm), followed by passive relaxation of the chest wall to its equilibrium position (Chapter 7). However, in more forceful breathing, for example, on exercise, expiration becomes active as a result of the activity of the expiratory cells. It should be noted that there is still not universal agreement on how the intrinsic rhythmicity of respiration is brought about by the medullary centers.

2. *Apneustic center* in the lower pons. This area is so named because if the brain of an experimental animal is sectioned just above this site, prolonged inspiratory gasps (apneuses) interrupted by transient expiratory efforts are seen. Apparently, the impulses from the center have an excitatory effect on the inspiratory area of the medulla, tending to prolong the ramp action potentials. Whether this apneustic center plays a role in normal human respiration is not known, although in some types of severe brain injury, this type of abnormal breathing is seen.

3. *Pneumotaxic center* in the upper pons. As indicated above, this area appears to "switch off" or inhibit inspiration and thus regulate inspiratory volume and, secondarily, respiratory rate. This has been demonstrated experimentally in animals by direct electrical stimulation of the pneumotaxic center. Some investigators believe that the role of this center is "fine tuning" of respiratory rhythm because a normal rhythm can exist in the absence of this center.

Cortex

Breathing is under voluntary control to a considerable extent, and the cortex can override the function of the brainstem within limits. It is not difficult to halve the arterial P_{CO_2} by hyperventilation, although the consequent alkalosis may cause tetany with contraction of the muscles of the hand and foot (carpopedal spasm). Halving the P_{CO_2} increases the arterial pH by about 0.2 unit (Figure 6.8).

Voluntary hypoventilation is more difficult. The duration of breath holding is limited by several factors, including the arterial P_{CO_2} and P_{O_2}. A preliminary period of hyperventilation increases breath-holding time, especially if oxygen is breathed. However, factors other than chemical are involved. This is shown by the observation that if at the breaking point of breathholding, a gas mixture is inhaled which *raises* the arterial P_{CO_2} and *lowers* the P_{O_2}, a further period of breathholding is possible.

Other Parts of the Brain

Other parts of the brain, such as the limbic system and hypo-thalamus, can alter the pattern of breathing, for example, in affective states such as rage and fear.

EFFECTORS

The muscles of respiration include the diaphragm, intercostal muscles, abdominal muscles, and accessory muscles such as the ster-nomastoids. The actions of these were described at the beginning of Chapter 7. In the context of the control of ventilation, it is crucially important that these various muscle groups work in a coordinated manner, and this is the responsibility of the central controller. There is evidence that some newborn children, particularly those that are premature, have uncoordinated respiratory muscle activity, especially during sleep. For example, the thoracic muscles may try to inspire while the abdominal muscles expire. This may be a factor in the "sudden infant death syndrome."

SENSORS

Central Chemoreceptors

A chemoreceptor is a receptor that responds to a change in the chemical composition of the blood or other fluid around it. The most important receptors involved in the minute-by-minute control of ventilation are those situated near the ventral surface of the medulla in the vicinity of the exit of the 9th and 10th nerves. In animals, local application of H^+ or dissolved CO_2 to this area stimulates breathing within a few seconds. At one time, it was thought that the medullary respiratory center itself was the site of action of CO_2, but it is now accepted that the chemoreceptors are anatomically separate. Some evidence suggests that they lie about 200–400 µm below the ventral surface of the medulla (Figure 8.2).

The central chemoreceptors are surrounded by brain extracellular fluid and respond to changes in its H^+ concentration. An increase in H^+ concentration stimulates ventilation while a decrease inhibits it. The composition of the extracellular fluid around the receptors is governed by the cerebrospinal fluid (CSF), local blood flow, and local metabolism.

Of these, the CSF is apparently the most important. It is separated from the blood by the blood-brain barrier, which is relatively impermeable to H^+ and HCO_3^- ions, although molecular CO_2 diffuses across it easily. When the blood P_{CO_2} rises, CO_2 diffuses into the CSF from the cerebral blood vessels, liberating H^+ ions which stimulate the chemoreceptors. Thus, the CO_2 level in blood regulates ventilation chiefly by its effect on the pH of the CSF. The resulting hyperventilation reduces the P_{CO_2} in the blood and therefore in the CSF. The cerebral vasodilation which accompanies an increased arterial P_{CO_2}

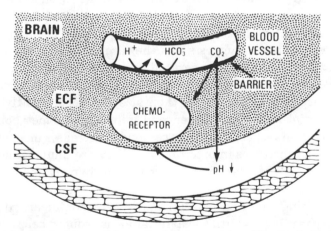

Figure 8.2. Environment of the central chemoreceptors. They are bathed in brain extracellular fluid (*ECF*) through which CO_2 easily diffuses from blood vessels to cerebrospinal fluid (*CSF*). The CO_2 reduces the CSF pH, thus stimulating the chemoreceptor. H^+ and HCO_3^- ions cannot easily cross the blood-brain barrier.

enhances diffusion of CO_2 into the CSF and the brain extracellular fluid.

The normal pH of the CSF is 7.32, and since the CSF contains much less protein than blood, it has a much lower buffering capacity. As a result, the change in CSF pH for a given change in P_{CO_2} is greater than in blood. If the CSF pH is displaced over a prolonged period, a compensatory change in HCO_3^- occurs as a result of transport across the blood-brain barrier. However, the CSF pH does not usually return to 7.32. The change in CSF pH occurs more promptly than the change of the pH of arterial blood by renal compensation (Figure 6.8), a process which takes 2–3 days. The partial resetting of the CSF pH in relation to blood pH results in its predominating influence on ventilation and arterial P_{CO_2}.

One example of these changes is a patient with chronic lung disease and CO_2 retention of long standing who may have a nearly normal CSF pH and, therefore, an abnormally low ventilation for his arterial P_{CO_2}. A similar situation is seen in normal subjects who are exposed to an atmosphere containing 3% CO_2 for some days.

Peripheral Chemoreceptors

These are located in the carotid bodies at the bifurcation of the common carotid arteries, and in the aortic bodies above and below the aortic arch. The carotid bodies are the most important in man. They contain glomus cells of two or more types which show an intense fluorescent staining because of their large content of dopamine. At one time these glomus cells were thought to be the chemoreceptors, but more recent work suggests that they are inhibitory interneurons and that the impulses are generated in the afferent terminals of the carotid sinus nerve (Figure 8.3A). The carotid bodies apparently have a very high blood flow for their size and, consequently, a very small arterial-venous O_2 difference in spite of a high metabolic rate.

The peripheral chemoreceptors respond to decreases in arterial P_{O_2} and pH, and increases in arterial P_{CO_2}. They are unique among tissues of the body in that their sensitivity to changes in arterial P_{O_2} begins around 500 mm Hg. Figure 8.3B shows that the relationship between firing rate and arterial P_{O_2} is very nonlinear; relatively little response occurs until the arterial P_{O_2} is reduced below 100 mm Hg, but then the rate rapidly increases. Because of their small arterial-venous difference, they respond to arterial rather than to venous P_{O_2}. The response of these receptors can be very fast; indeed, their discharge rate can alter during the respiratory cycle as a result

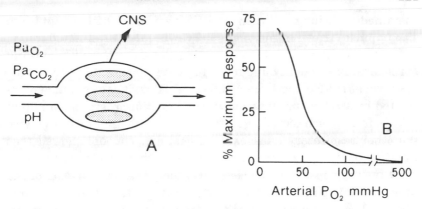

Figure 8.3. *A* shows a carotid body which responds to changes of P_{O_2}, P_{CO_2}, and pH in arterial blood. Impulses travel to the central nervous system (*CNS*) through Hering's nerve. *B* shows the nonlinear response to arterial P_{O_2}. Note that the maximum response occurs below a P_{O_2} of 50 mm Hg.

of the small cyclic changes in blood gases. The peripheral chemoreceptors are responsible for all the increase of ventilation that occurs in man in response to arterial hypoxemia. Indeed, in the absence of these receptors, severe hypoxemia depresses respiration, presumably through a direct effect on the respiratory centers. Complete loss of hypoxic ventilatory drive has been shown in patients with bilateral carotid body resection.

The response of the peripheral chemoreceptors to arterial P_{CO_2} is much less important than that of the central chemoreceptors. For example, when a normal subject is given a CO_2 mixture to breathe, less than 20% of the ventilatory response can be attributed to the peripheral chemoreceptors. However, their response is more rapid, and they may be useful in matching ventilation to abrupt changes in P_{CO_2}.

In man, the carotid but not the aortic bodies respond to a fall in arterial pH. This occurs regardless of whether the cause is respiratory or metabolic. Interaction of the various stimuli occurs. Thus, increases in chemoreceptor activity in response to decreases in arterial P_{O_2} are potentiated by increases in P_{CO_2} and, in the carotid bodies, by decreases in pH.

Lung Receptors

1. Pulmonary Stretch Receptors

These are believed to lie within airway smooth muscle. They discharge in response to distention of the lung, and their activity is sustained with lung inflation, that is, they show little adaptation. The impulses travel in the vagus nerve via large myelinated fibers.

The main reflex effect of stimulating these receptors is a slowing of respiratory frequency due to an increase in expiratory time. This is known as the Hering-Breuer inflation reflex. It can be well demonstrated in a rabbit preparation where the diaphragm has a slip of muscle from which recordings can be made without interfering with the other respiratory muscles. Classical experiments showed that inflation of the lungs tended to inhibit further inspiratory muscle activity. The opposite response is also seen, that is, deflation of the lungs tends to initiate inspiratory activity (deflation reflex). Thus these reflexes can provide a self-regulatory mechanism or negative feedback.

The Hering-Breuer reflexes were once thought to play a major role in ventilation by determining the rate and depth of breathing. This could be done by using the information from these stretch receptors to modulate the "switching off" mechanism in the medulla. Thus, bilateral vagotomy which removes the input of these receptors causes slow, deep breathing in most animals. However, more recent work indicates that the reflexes are largely inactive in adult man unless the tidal volume exceeds 1 liter, as in exercise. It has been shown that transient bilateral blockade of the vagi by local anesthesia in awake man does not change either breathing rate or volume. There is some evidence that these reflexes may be more important in newborn babies.

2. Irritant Receptors

These are thought to lie between airway epithelial cells, and they are stimulated by noxious gases, cigarette smoke, inhaled dusts, and cold air. The impulses travel up the vagus in myelinated fibers, and the reflex effects include bronchoconstriction and hyperpnea. Some physiologists prefer to call these receptors "rapidly adapting receptors" because they show rapid adaptation and are apparently involved in additional mechanoreceptor functions, as well as responding to noxious stimuli on the airway walls. It is possible that irritant receptors play a role in the bronchoconstriction of asthma attacks as a result of their response to released histamine.

3. J Receptors

The term "juxta-capillary," or J, is used because the receptors are believed to be in the alveolar walls close to the capillaries. The evidence for this location is that they respond very quickly to chemicals injected into the pulmonary circulation. The impulses pass up the vagus nerve in slowly conducting nonmyelinated fibers and can result in rapid, shallow breathing, although intense stimulation causes apnea. There is evidence that engorgement of pulmonary capillaries and increases in the interstitial fluid volume of the alveolar wall activate these receptors. They may play a role in the dyspnea (sensation of difficulty in breathing) associated with left heart failure and interstitial lung disease.

Other Receptors

1. Nose and Upper Airway Receptors

The nose, nasopharynx, larynx, and trachea contain receptors that respond to mechanical and chemical stimulation. These are an extension of the irritant receptors described above. Various reflex responses have been described including sneezing, coughing, and bronchoconstriction. Laryngeal spasm may occur if the larynx is irritated mechanically, for example, during insertion of an endotracheal tube with insufficient local anesthesia.

2. Joint and Muscle Receptors

Impulses from moving limbs are believed to be part of the stimulus to ventilation during exercise, especially in the early stages.

3. Gamma System

Many muscles, including the intercostal muscles and diaphragm, contain muscle spindles which sense elongation of the muscle. This information is used to reflexly control the strength of contraction. These receptors may be involved in the sensation of dyspnea, which occurs when unusually large respiratory efforts are required to move the lung and chest wall, for example, because of airway obstruction.

4. Arterial Baroreceptors

Increase in arterial blood pressure can cause reflex hypoventilation or apnea through stimulation of the aortic and carotid sinus baroreceptors. Conversely, a decrease in blood pressure may result in hyperventilation. The pathways of these reflexes are largely unknown.

5. Pain and Temperature

Stimulation of many afferent nerves can bring about changes in ventilation. Pain often causes a period of apnea followed by hyperventilation. Heating of the skin may result in hyperventilation.

INTEGRATED RESPONSES

Now that we have looked at the various units that make up the respiratory control system (Figure 8.1), it is useful to consider the overall responses of the system to changes in the arterial CO_2, O_2, and pH, and to exercise.

Response to Carbon Dioxide

The most important factor in the control of ventilation under normal conditions is the P_{CO_2} of the arterial blood. The sensitivity of this control is remarkable. In the course of daily activity with periods of rest and exercise, the arterial P_{CO_2} is probably held to within 3 mm Hg. During sleep it may rise a little more.

The ventilatory response to CO_2 is normally measured by having the subject inhale CO_2 mixtures or rebreathe from a bag so that the inspired P_{CO_2} gradually rises. In one technique the subject rebreathes from a bag which is prefilled with 7% CO_2 and 93% O_2. As he rebreathes, he adds metabolic CO_2 to the bag, but the O_2 concentration remains relatively high. In such a procedure the P_{CO_2} of the bag gas increases at the rate of about 4 mm Hg/min.

Figure 8.4 shows the results of experiments carried out in which the inspired mixture was adjusted to yield a constant alveolar P_{O_2}. (In this type of experiment on normal subjects, alveolar end-tidal P_{O_2} and P_{CO_2} are generally taken to reflect the arterial levels.) It can be seen that with a normal P_{O_2} the ventilation increases by about 2–3 liters/min for each 1 mm Hg rise in P_{CO_2}. Lowering the P_{O_2} produces two effects: there is a higher ventilation for a given P_{CO_2} and, also, the slope of the line becomes steeper. There is considerable variation between subjects.

Another way of measuring respiratory drive is to record the inspiratory pressure during a brief period of airway occlusion. The subject breathes through a mouthpiece attached to a valve box, and the inspiratory port is provided with a shutter. This is closed during an expiration (the subject being unaware), so that the first part of his next inspiration is against an occluded airway. The shutter is opened after about 0.5 sec. The pressure generated during the first 0.1 sec

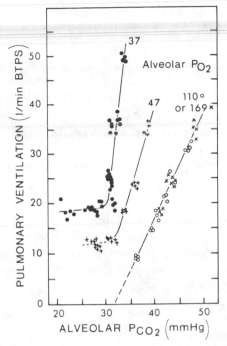

Figure 8.4. Ventilatory response to CO_2. Each curve of total ventilation against alveolar P_{CO_2} is for a different alveolar P_{O_2}. In this study, no difference was found between an alveolar P_{O_2} of 110 mm Hg and one of 169 mm Hg, though some investigators have found that the slope of the line is slightly less at the higher P_{O_2}. (From M Nielsen and H Smith: *Acta Physiol Scand* 24:293, 1951.)

of attempted inspiration (known as $P_{0.1}$) is taken as a measure of respiratory center output. This is largely unaffected by the mechanical properties of the respiratory system, although it may be influenced by lung volume. This method can be used to study the respiratory sensitivity to CO_2 hypoxia, and other variables as well.

A reduction in arterial P_{CO_2} is very effective in reducing the stimulus to ventilation. For example, if the reader hyperventilates voluntarily for a few seconds, he will find that he has no urge to breathe for a short period. An anesthetized patient will frequently stop breathing for a minute or so if he is first overventilated by the anesthesiologist.

The ventilatory response to CO_2 is reduced by sleep, increasing age, and genetic, racial, and personality factors. Trained athletes and divers tend to have a low CO_2 sensitivity. Various drugs depress the respiratory center, including morphine and barbiturates. Patients who have taken an overdose of one of these drugs often have marked hypoventilation. The ventilatory response to CO_2 is also reduced if the work of breathing is increased. This can be demonstrated by having normal subjects breathe through a narrow tube. The neural output of the respiratory center is not reduced, but it is not so effective in producing ventilation. The abnormally small ventilatory response to CO_2 and the CO_2 retention in some patients with lung disease can be partly explained by the same mechanism. In such patients, reducing the airway resistance with bronchodilators often increases their ventilatory response. There is also some evidence that the sensitivity of the respiratory center is reduced in these patients.

As we have seen, the main stimulus to increase ventilation when the arterial P_{CO_2} rises comes from the central chemoreceptors, which respond to the increased H^+ concentration of the brain extracellular fluid near the receptors. An additional stimulus comes from the peripheral chemoreceptors, because of both the rise in arterial P_{CO_2} and the fall in pH.

Response to Oxygen

The way in which a reduction of P_{O_2} in arterial blood stimulates ventilation can be studied by having a subject breathe hypoxic gas mixtures. The end-tidal P_{O_2} and P_{CO_2} are used as a measure of the arterial values. Figure 8.5 shows that when the alveolar P_{CO_2} is kept at about 36 mm Hg (by altering the inspired mixture), the alveolar P_{O_2} can be reduced to the vicinity of 50 mm Hg before any appreciable increase in ventilation occurs. Raising the P_{CO_2} increases the ventilation at any P_{O_2} (compare Figure 8.4). Note that when the P_{CO_2} is increased, a reduction in P_{O_2} below 100 mm Hg causes some stimulation of ventilation, unlike the situation when the P_{CO_2} is normal. Thus, the combined effects of both stimuli exceed the sum of each stimulus given separately, and this is referred to as interaction between the high CO_2 and low O_2 stimuli. Large differences in response occur between individual subjects.

Since the P_{O_2} can normally be reduced so far without evoking a ventilatory response, the role of this hypoxic stimulus in the day-by-day control of ventilation is small. However, on ascent to high altitude, a large increase in ventilation occurs in response to the hypoxia (see Chapter 9).

In some patients with severe lung disease, the hypoxic drive to ventilation becomes very important. These patients have chronic

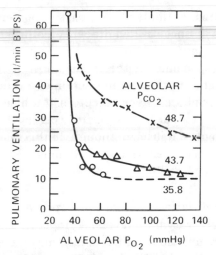

Figure 8.5. Hypoxic response curves. Note that when the P_{CO_2} is 36 mm Hg, almost no increase in ventilation occurs until the P_{O_2} is reduced to about 50 mm Hg. (Modified from HH Loeschke and KH Gertz: *Arch Ges Physiol* 267:460, 1958.)

CO_2 retention, and the pH of their brain extracellular fluid has returned to near normal in spite of a raised P_{CO_2}. Thus, they have lost most of their increase in the CO_2 stimulus to ventilation. In addition, the initial depression of blood pH has been nearly abolished by renal compensation so that there is little pH stimulation of the peripheral chemoreceptors (see below). Under these conditions, the arterial hypoxemia becomes the chief stimulus to ventilation. If such a patient is given a high O_2 mixture to breathe to relieve his hypoxemia, his ventilation may become grossly depressed. His ventilatory state is best monitored by measuring his arterial P_{CO_2}.

As we have seen, hypoxemia reflexly stimulates ventilation by its action on the carotid and aortic body chemoreceptors. It has no action on the central chemoreceptors; indeed, in the absence of peripheral chemoreceptors, hypoxemia depresses respiration. However, prolonged hypoxemia can cause mild cerebral acidosis which in turn can stimulate ventilation.

Response to pH

A reduction in arterial blood pH stimulates ventilation. In practice, it is often difficult to separate the ventilatory response resulting from a fall in pH from that caused by an accompanying rise in P_{CO_2}. However, in experimental animals in whom it is possible to reduce the pH at a constant P_{CO_2}, the stimulus to ventilation can be convincingly demonstrated. Patients with a partly compensated metabolic acidosis (such as in uncontrolled diabetes mellitus) who have a low pH and low P_{CO_2} (Figures 6.8 and 6.9) show an increased ventilation. Indeed, this is responsible for the reduced P_{CO_2}.

As we have seen, the chief site of action of a reduced arterial pH is probably the peripheral chemoreceptors. It is also possible that the central chemoreceptors or the respiratory center itself is affected by a change in blood pH if it is large enough. In this case the blood-brain barrier becomes partly permeable to H^+ ions.

Response to Exercise

On exercise, ventilation increases promptly and during strenuous exertion may reach very high levels. A fit young man who attains a maximum O_2 consumption of 4 liters/min may have a total ventilation of 120 liters/min, that is, about 15 times his resting level. This increase in ventilation closely matches the increase in O_2 uptake and CO_2 output. It is remarkable that the cause of the increased ventilation on exercise remains largely unknown.

The arterial P_{CO_2} does not increase during exercise; indeed, during severe exercise it typically falls slightly. The arterial P_{O_2} usually increases slightly, although it may fall at very high work levels. The arterial pH remains nearly constant for moderate exercise, although during heavy exercise it falls because of the liberation of lactic acid through anaerobic glycolysis. It is clear, therefore, that none of the mechanisms we have discussed so far can account for the large increase in ventilation observed during light to moderate exercise.

Other stimuli have been suggested. *Passive movement of the limbs* stimulates ventilation in both anesthetized animals and awake man. This is a reflex with receptors presumably located in joints or muscles. It is probably responsible for the abrupt increase in ventilation which occurs during the first few seconds of exercise. One hypothesis is that *oscillations in arterial P_{O_2} and P_{CO_2}* may stimulate the peripheral chemoreceptors even though the mean level remains unaltered. These fluctuations are caused by the periodic nature of ventilation and increase when the tidal volume rises, as on exercise. Another theory is that the central chemoreceptors increase ventilation to hold the *arterial P_{CO_2} constant* by some kind of servomechanism, just as the thermostat can control a furnace with little change in temperature. The objection that the arterial P_{CO_2} often *falls* on exercise is countered by the assertion that the preferred level of P_{CO_2} is reset in some way. Proponents of this theory believe that the ventilatory response to inhaled CO_2 may not be a reliable guide to what happens on exercise.

Yet another hypothesis is that ventilation is linked in some way to the additional CO_2 *load* presented to the lungs in the mixed venous blood during exercise. In animal experiments, an increase in this load produced either by infusing CO_2 into the venous blood or by increasing venous return has been shown to correlate well with ventilation. However, a problem with this hypothesis is that no suitable receptor has been found.

Additional factors which have been suggested include the *increase in body temperature* during exercise which stimulates ventilation and *impulses from the motor cortex*. However, none of the theories proposed so far is completely satisfactory.

ABNORMAL PATTERNS OF BREATHING

Subjects with severe hypoxemia often exhibit a striking pattern of periodic breathing known as *Cheyne-Stokes respiration*. This is characterized by periods of apnea of 10–20 sec, separated by approximately equal periods of hyperventilation when the tidal volume gradually waxes and then wanes. This pattern is frequently seen at high altitude, especially at night during sleep. It is also found in some patients with severe heart disease or brain damage.

The pattern can be reproduced in experimental animals by lengthening the distance through which blood travels on its way to the brain from the lung. Under these conditions, there is a long delay before the central chemoreceptors sense the alteration in PO_{CO_2} caused by a change in ventilation. As a result, the respiratory center hunts for the equilibrium condition, always overshooting it. However, not all instances of Cheyne-Stokes respiration can be explained on this basis.

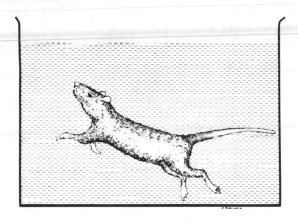

chapter 9

Respiratory Physiology in Unusual Environments

*how gas exchange is accomplished at
low and high pressures and at birth*

The lung serves as our principal physiological link with the environment we live in; its surface area is some 30 times that of the skin. Man's urge to climb higher and diver deeper puts the respiratory system under great stress, although these situations are minor insults compared with the process of being born! In this chapter we look at some of the problems of unusual environments which often throw light on normal pulmonary function.

HIGH ALTITUDE

The barometric pressure decreases with distance above the earth's surface in an approximately exponential manner (Figure 9.1). The pressure at 5,500 m (18,000 ft) is only one-half the normal 760 mm

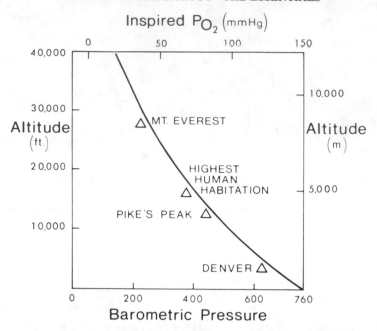

Figure 9.1. Relationship between altitude and barometric pressure. Note that at 1,520 m (5,000 ft) (Denver), the P_{O_2} of moist inspired gas is about 130 mm Hg, but is only 43 mm Hg on the summit of Mount Everest.

Hg, so the P_{O_2} of moist inspired gas is $(380 - 47) \times 0.2093 = 70$ mm Hg (47 mm Hg is the partial pressure of water vapor at body temperature—see p. 2). At the summit of Mount Everest (altitude 8,848 m or 29,028 ft), the inspired P_{O_2} is only 43 mm Hg. At 19,200 m (63,000 ft), the barometric pressure is 47 mm Hg so that the inspired P_{O_2} is zero.

In spite of the hypoxia associated with high altitude, some 15 million people live at elevations over 3,050 m (10,000 ft), and permanent residents live higher than 4,900 m (16,000 ft) in the Andes. A remarkable degree of acclimatization occurs when man ascends to these altitudes; indeed, climbers have lived for several days at altitudes which would cause unconsciousness within a few seconds in the absence of acclimatization.

Hyperventilation

One of the most useful responses to high altitude is hyperventilation. Its physiological value can be seen by considering the alveolar gas equation (see p. 54) for a climber on the summit of Mount

Everest. If his alveolar P_{CO_2} were 40 and respiratory exchange ratio 1, his alveolar P_{O_2} would be $43 - (40/1)^* = 3$ mm Hg! However, by increasing his ventilation fourfold, and thus reducing his P_{CO_2} to 10 mm Hg (see p. 53), he can raise his alveolar P_{O_2} to $43 - 10 = 33$ mm Hg. Typically the arterial P_{CO_2} in permanent residents at 4,600 m (15,000 ft) is about 33 mm Hg.

The cause of the hyperventilation is hypoxic stimulation of the peripheral chemoreceptors. The resulting low arterial P_{CO_2} and alkalosis tend to work against this increase in ventilation, but after a day or so, the cerebrospinal fluid (CSF) pH is brought partly back by movement of bicarbonate out of the CSF, and after 2 or 3 days, the pH of the arterial blood is returned to near normal by renal excretion of bicarbonate. These brakes on ventilation are then reduced, and it increases further. Interestingly, people born at high altitude have a diminished ventilatory response to hypoxia which is only slowly corrected by subsequent residence at sea level. Conversely, those born at sea level who move to high altitudes retain their hypoxic response intact for a long time. Apparently, therefore, this ventilatory response is determined very early in life.

Polycythemia

Another apparently valuable feature of acclimatization to high altitude is an increase in the red blood cell concentration of the blood. The resulting rise in hemoglobin concentration, and therefore O_2 carrying capacity, means that although the arterial P_{O_2} and O_2 saturation are diminished, the O_2 content of the arterial blood may be normal or even above normal. For example, in permanent residents at 4,600 (15,000 ft) in the Peruvian Andes the arterial P_{O_2} is only 45 mm Hg, and the corresponding arterial O_2 saturation is only 81%. Ordinarily this would considerably decrease the arterial O_2 content, but because of the polycythemia, the hemoglobin concentration is increased from 15 to 19.8 gm/100 ml, giving an arterial O_2 concentration of 22.4 ml/100 ml, which is above the normal sea level value. The polycythemia also tends to maintain the P_{O_2} of mixed venous blood and typically in Andean natives living at 4,600 (15,000 ft), this P_{O_2} is only 7 mm Hg below normal (Figure 9.2). The stimulus for the increased production of red blood cells is hypoxemia which releases hemopoietin from the kidney which in turn stimulates the

---

*When R = 1, the correction factor shown on p. 54 vanishes.

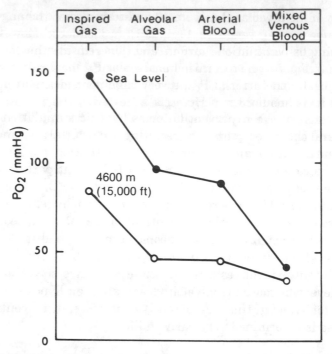

Figure 9.2. Scheme of the P_{O_2} levels from inspired air to mixed venous blood at sea level and in residents at an altitude of 4,600 m (15,000 ft). Note that in spite of the much lower inspired P_{O_2} at altitude, the P_{O_2} of the mixed venous blood is only 7 mm Hg lower. (From A Hurtado: In Dill DB: *Handbook of Physiology, Adaptation to the Environment.* Washington, DC, American Physiological Society, 1964.)

bone marrow. Polycythemia is also seen in many patients with chronic hypoxemia caused by lung or heart disease.

Although the polycythemia of high altitude increases the O_2-carrying capacity of the blood, it also raises the blood viscosity. This can be deleterious, and some physiologists have argued that the marked polycythemia which is sometimes seen is an inappropriate response.

Other Features of Acclimatization

These include a *shift to the right of the O_2 dissociation curve* which results in a better unloading of O_2 in venous blood at a given P_{O_2}. The cause of the shift is an increase in concentration of 2,3-diphosphoglycerate which develops primarily because of the respiratory alkalosis. However, the righward shift interferes with the loading of O_2 in the lung, and some recent work suggests that a leftward shift is actually more advantageous. There is evidence that the *number of capillaries per unit volume* in peripheral tissues increases, and also that changes occur in the *oxidative enzymes* inside the cells. The *maximum breathing capacity* increases because the air is less dense (see p. 107), and this assists the very high ventilations (up to 200 liters/min) which occur on exercise. However, the maximum O_2 uptake declines rapidly above 4,600 m (15,000 ft). This is corrected to a large extent (though not completely) if 100% O_2 is breathed.

An important feature is the *pulmonary vasoconstriction* which occurs in response to alveolar hypoxia (see p. 43). As a consequence, the pulmonary arterial pressure rises, as does the work done by the right heart. This is exaggerated by the polycythemia which raises the viscosity of the blood. Hypertrophy of the right heart is seen with characteristic changes in the electrocardiogram. There seems to be no physiological advantage in this response, except that the topographical distribution of blood flow becomes more uniform (see p. 40). The pulmonary hypertension is sometimes associated with pulmonary edema, although the pulmonary venous pressure is normal. The mechanism for this is obscure, but one hypothesis is that the arteriolar vasoconstriction is uneven and leakage occurs in unprotected, damaged capillaries. The edema fluid has a high protein concentration, indicating that the permeability of the capillaries is increased.

Newcomers to high altitude frequently complain of headache, fatigue, dizziness, palpitations, nausea, loss of appetite, and insomnia. This is known as *acute mountain sickness* and is attributable to the hypoxemia and alkalosis. Long-term residents sometimes develop an ill-defined syndrome characterized by fatigue, reduced exercise tolerance, severe hypoxemia, and marked polycythemia. This is called *chronic mountain sickness*.

O_2 TOXICITY

The usual problem is getting enough O_2 into the body, but it is possible to have too much. When high concentrations of O_2 are breathed for many hours, damage to the lung may occur. If guinea pigs are placed in 100% O_2 at atmospheric pressure for 48 hours, they develop pulmonary edema. The first pathological changes are seen in the endothelial cells of the pulmonary capillaries (see Figure 1.1). It is (perhaps fortunately) difficult to administer very high concentrations of O_2 to patients, but evidence of impaired gas exchange has

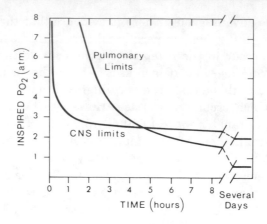

Figure 9.3. Relationship between P_{O_2} and exposure time responsible for O_2 toxicity. (From CJ Lambertsen: In JR DiPalma: *Drill's Pharmacology in Medicine*. New York, McGraw-Hill, 1971.)

been demonstrated after 30 hours of inhalation of 100% O_2 (Figure 9.3). Normal volunteers who breathe 100% O_2 at atmospheric pressure for 24 hours complain of substernal distress which is aggravated by deep breathing, and they develop a diminution of vital capacity of 500–800 ml. This is probably caused by absorption atelectasis (see below).

Another hazard of breathing 100% O_2 is seen in premature infants who develop blindness because of retrolental fibroplasia, that is, fibrous tissue formation behind the lens. Here the mechanism is local vasoconstriction caused by the high P_{O_2} in the incubator and it can be avoided if the arterial P_{O_2} is kept below 140 mm Hg.

Absorption Atelectasis

This is another danger of breathing 100% O_2. Suppose that an airway is obstructed by mucus (Figure 9.4). The total pressure in the trapped gas is close to 760 mm Hg (it may be a few mm Hg less as it is absorbed because of elastic forces in the lung). But the sum of the partial pressures in the venous blood is far less than 760 mm Hg. This is because the P_{O_2} of the venous blood remains relatively low, even when O_2 is breathed. In fact the rise in O_2 *concentration* of arterial and venous blood when O_2 is breathed will be the same if cardiac output remains unchanged (see p. 39), but because of the shape of the O_2 dissociation curve (Figure 6.1), the increase in venous P_{O_2} is only about 10–15 mm Hg. Thus, since the sum of the partial

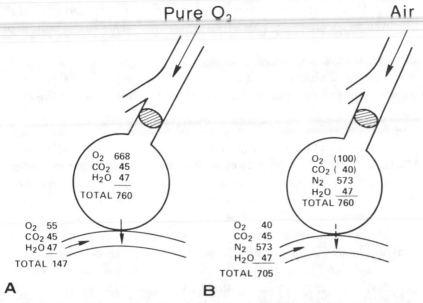

Figure 9.4. Reasons for atelectasis of alveoli beyond blocked airways (A) when O_2 and (B) when air is breathed. Note that in both cases, the sum of the gas partial pressures in the mixed venous blood is less than in the alveoli. In B, the P_{O_2} and P_{CO_2} are shown in parentheses because these values change with time. However, the total alveolar pressure remains within a few mm Hg of 760.

pressures in the alveolar gas greatly exceeds that in the venous blood, gas diffuses into the blood, and rapid collapse of the alveoli occurs. Reopening such an atelectatic area may be difficult because of surface tension effects in such small units (see Figure 7.4).

Absorption collapse also occurs in a blocked region, even when air is breathed, although here the process is slower. Figure 9.4B shows that again the sum of the partial pressures in venous blood is less than 760 mm Hg because the fall in P_{O_2} from arterial to venous blood is much greater than the rise in P_{CO_2} (this is a reflection of the steeper slope of the CO_2 compared with the O_2 dissociation curve—see Figure 6.7A). Since the total gas pressure in the alveoli is near 760 mm Hg, absorption is inevitable. Actually the changes in the alveolar partial pressures during absorption are somewhat complicated, but it can be shown that the rate of collapse is limited by the rate of absorption of N_2. Since this gas has a low solubility, its presence acts as a "splint" which, as it were, supports the alveoli and delays collapse. Even relatively small concentrations of N_2 in alveolar gas have a useful splinting effect. Nevertheless, postoperative atelectasis is a common problem in patients who are treated with high O_2 mixtures. Collapse is particularly likely to occur at the bottom of the lung where the parenchyma is least well expanded (Figure 7.8) or the airways are actually closed (Figure 7.9). This same basic mechanism of absorption is responsible for the gradual disappearance of a pneumothorax, or a gas pocket introduced under the skin.

SPACE FLIGHT

The absence of gravity causes a number of physiological changes which are poorly understood at the present time. Some of these affect the lung. The distribution of ventilation and blood flow become more uniform, with a small corresponding improvement in gas exchange (see Figures 5.8 and 5.10). The deposition of inhaled aerosol is altered because of the absence of sedimentation (p. 141). In addition, central blood volume initially increases because blood does not pool in the legs, and this apparently causes a diuresis. Cardiovascular deconditioning occurs with postural hypotension on return to earth. Decalcification of bone and muscle degeneration may occur, presumably through disuse. There is a small reduction in red cell mass which is as yet unexplained. Space sickness (space adaptation syndrome) is a serious operational problem.

INCREASED PRESSURE

During diving the pressure increases by 1 atmosphere for every 10 m (33 ft) of descent. Pressure by itself is relatively innocuous,† as long as it is balanced. However, if a gas cavity such as the lung, middle ear, or intracranial sinus fails to communicate with the outside, the pressure difference may cause compression on descent or overexpansion on ascent. For example, it is very important for a diver to exhale as he ascends in order to prevent overinflation and possible rupture of his lung. The increased density of the gas at depth increases the work of breathing (see p. 107). This may result in CO_2 retention, especially on exercise.

Decompression Sickness

During diving the high partial pressure of N_2 force this poorly soluble gas into solution in body tissues. This particularly occurs in

---

† At pressure of hundreds of atmospheres, chemical reactions are affected. For example, the O_2 dissociation curve is displaced.

fat, which has a relatively high N_2 solubility. However, the blood supply of adipose tissue is meager, and the blood can carry little N_2. In addition the gas diffuses slowly because of its low solubility. As a result, equilibration of N_2 between the tissues and the environment takes hours.

During ascent, N_2 is slowly removed from the tissues. If decompression is unduly rapid, bubbles of gaseous N_2 form, just as CO_2 is released when a bottle of champagne is opened. Some bubbles can occur without physiological disturbances, but large numbers of bubbles cause pain, especially in the region of joints ("bends"). In severe cases there may be neurological disturbances such as deafness, impaired vision, and even paralysis caused by bubbles in the central nervous system (CNS) which obstruct blood flow.

The treatment of decompression sickness is by recompression. This reduces the volume of the bubbles and forces them back into solution, and often results in a dramatic reduction of symptoms. Prevention is by careful decompression in a series of regulated steps. There are schedules which are based partly on theory and partly on experience and show how rapidly a diver can come up with little risk of developing bends. A short but very deep dive may require hours of gradual decompression. Recent work shows that bubble formation during ascent is very common. Therefore the aim of the decompression schedules is to prevent the bubbles from growing too large.

The risk of decompression sickness following very deep dives can be reduced if a helium-O_2 mixture is breathed during the dive. Helium is about one-half as soluble as N_2 so that less is dissolved in tissues. In addition, it has one-seventh of the molecular weight of N_2 and therefore diffuses more rapidly through tissue (Figure 3.1). Both these factors reduce the risk of bends. Another advantage of a helium-O_2 mixture for divers is its low density, which reduces the work of breathing. Pure O_2 or enriched O_2 mixtures cannot be used at depth because of the dangers of O_2 toxicity (see below).

Inert Gas Narcosis

Although we often think of N_2 as a physiologically inert gas, at high partial pressures it affects the CNS. At a depth of about 50 m (160 ft) there is a feeling of euphoria (not unlike that following a martini or two), and divers have been known to offer their mouthpieces to fish! At higher partial pressures, loss of coordination and eventually coma may develop.

The mechanism of action is not understood but may be related to the high fat : water solubility of N_2 which is a general property of anesthetic agents. Other gases such as helium and hydrogen can be used at much greater depths without narcotic effects.

O_2 Toxicity

We saw earlier (p. 135) that inhalation of 100% O_2 at 1 atmosphere can damage the lung. Another form of O_2 toxicity is stimulation of the CNS, leading to convulsions, when the P_{O_2} considerably exceeds 760 mm Hg. The convulsions may be preceded by premonitory symptoms such as nausea, ringing in the ears, and twitching of the face.

The likelihood of convulsions depends on the inspired P_{O_2} and the duration of exposure (Figure 9.3), and it is increased if the subject is exercising. At a P_{O_2} of 4 atmospheres, convulsions frequently occur within 30 minutes. For increasingly deep dives, the O_2 concentration is progressively reduced to avoid toxic effects and may eventually be less than 1% for a normal inspired P_{O_2}! The amateur scuba diver should *never* fill his tanks with O_2 because of the danger of a convulsion underwater. However, pure O_2 is sometimes used by the military for shallow dives because a closed breathing circuit with a CO_2 absorber leaves no tell-tale bubbles. The biochemical basis for the deleterious effects of a high P_{O_2} on the CNS is not fully understood but is probably the inactivation of certain enzymes, especially dehydrogenases containing sulfhydryl groups.

Hyperbaric O_2 Therapy

Increasing the arterial P_{O_2} to a very high level is useful in some clinical situations. One is severe CO poisoning where most of the hemoglobin is bound to CO and is therefore unavailable to carry O_2. By raising the inspired P_{O_2} to 3 atmospheres in special chambers, the amount of dissolved O_2 in arterial blood can be increased to about 6 ml/100 ml (Figure 6.1), and thus the needs of the tissues can be met without functioning hemoglobin. Occasionally, an anemic crisis is managed in this way. Hyperbaric O_2 is also useful for treating gas gangrene because the organism cannot live in a high P_{O_2} environment. A hyperbaric chamber is also useful for treating decompression sickness.

Fire and explosions are serious hazards of a 100% O_2 atmosphere, especially at increased pressure. For this reason, O_2 in a pressure chamber is given by mask, and the chamber itself is filled with air.

POLLUTED ATMOSPHERES‡

Unhappily, a polluted atmosphere is becoming less and less of an unusual environment as the number of motor vehicles and industries increases. The chief pollutants are various nitrogen oxides, the oxides of sulfur SO_2 and SO_3, ozone, carbon monoxide, various hydrocarbons, and particulate matter. Of these, nitrogen oxides, hydrocarbons, and CO are produced in considerable quantities by the internal combustion engine, the sulfur oxides mainly come from fossil fuel power stations, and ozone is chiefly formed in the atmosphere by the action of sunlight on nitrogen oxides and hydrocarbons. The concentration of atmospheric pollutants is greatly increased by a temperature inversion which prevents the normal escape of the warm surface air to the upper atmosphere.

Nitrogen oxides cause inflammation of the upper respiratory tract and eye irritation, and they are responsible for the yellow haze of smog. Sulfur oxides and ozone also cause bronchial inflammation, and ozone in high concentrations can produce pulmonary edema. The danger of CO is its propensity to tie up hemoglobin (see p. 74), and cyclic hydrocarbons are potentially carcinogenic. Both these pollutants exist in tobacco smoke, which is inhaled in far higher concentrations than any atmospheric pollution. There is evidence that some pollutants act synergistically, that is, their combined action exceeds the sum of their individual actions, but more work is required in this area.

Many pollutants exist as *aerosols*, that is, very small particles that remain suspended in the air. When an aerosol is inhaled, its fate depends on the size of the particles. Large particles are removed by *impaction* in the nose and pharynx. This means that the particles are unable to turn the corners rapidly because of their inertia, and they impinge on the wet mucosa and are trapped. Medium-sized particles deposit in small airways and elsewhere because of their weight. This is called *sedimentation* and occurs especially where the flow velocity is suddenly reduced because of the enormous increase in combined airway cross-section (Figure 1.5). For this reason deposition is heavy in the terminal and respiratory bronchioles, and this region of a coal miner's lung shows a heavy dust concentration. The smallest particles (less than 0.1 micron in diameter) reach the alveoli, where

‡For a more detailed account, see JB West: *Pulmonary Pathophysiology—the essentials,* ed 3. Baltimore, Williams & Wilkins, 1987, p 134.

some deposition occurs through *diffusion* to the walls. Many small particles are not deposited at all but are exhaled with the next breath.

Once deposited, most of the particles are removed by various clearance mechanisms. Particles which deposit on bronchial walls are swept up the moving staircase of mucus which is propelled by cilia, and they are either swallowed or expectorated. However, the ciliary action can be paralyzed by inhaled irritants. Particles which are deposited in the alveoli are chiefly engulfed by macrophages which leave via the blood or lymphatics.

LIQUID BREATHING

It is possible for mammals to survive for some hours breathing liquid instead of air. This was first shown with mice in saline in which the O_2 concentration was increased by exposure to 100% O_2 at 8 atmospheres pressure. Subsequently, mice, rats, and dogs have survived a period of breathing fluorocarbon exposed to pure O_2 at 1 atmosphere. This liquid has a high solubility for both O_2 and CO_2. The animals successfully returned to air breathing.

Because liquids have a much higher density and viscosity than air, the work of breathing is enormously increased. However, adequate oxygenation of the arterial blood can be obtained if the inspired concentration is raised sufficiently. Interestingly, a serious problem is eliminating CO_2. We saw on p. 6 that diffusion within the airways is chiefly responsible for the gas exchange that occurs between the alveoli and the terminal or respiratory bronchioles, where bulk flow takes over. Because the diffusion rates of gases in liquid are many orders of magnitude slower than in the gas phase, this means that a large partial pressure difference for CO_2 between the alveoli and terminal bronchioles must be maintained. Animals breathing liquid, therefore, commonly develop CO_2 retention and acidosis. Note that the diffusion pressure for O_2 can always be raised by increasing the inspired P_{O_2}, but this option is not available to help eliminate CO_2.

PERINATAL RESPIRATION

Placental Gas Exchange

During fetal life, gas exchange takes place through the placenta. Maternal blood enters from the uterine arteries and surges into small spaces called the intervillous sinusoids. Fetal blood is supplied through the umbilical arteries to capillary loops which protrude into the intervillous spaces. Gas exchange occurs across the blood-blood barrier approximately 3.5 microns thick.

This arrangement is much less efficient for gas exchange than the adult lung. Maternal blood apparently swirls around the sinusoids somewhat haphazardly, and there are probably large differences in P_{O_2} within these blood spaces. Contrast this situation with the air-filled alveoli where gaseous diffusion stirs up the alveolar contents. The result is that the P_{O_2} of the fetal blood leaving the placenta in the umbilical vein (UV) is only about 30 mm Hg (Figure 9.5).

This umbilical venous blood enters the inferior vena cava (IVC) via the ductus venosus (DV). This also receives portal vein (PV)

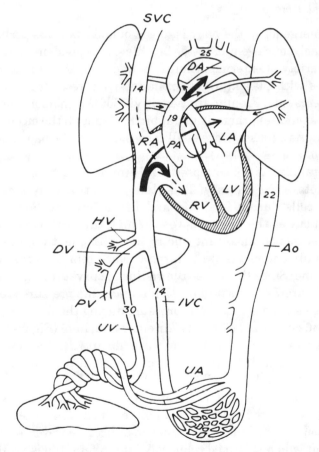

Figure 9.5.   Blood circulation in the human fetus. The numbers show the P_{O_2} of the blood in mm Hg. See text for details. (From JH Comroe: *Physiology of Respiration*, ed 2. Chicago, Year Book, 1974.)

blood which depresses the O_2 saturation further. Some of this blood enters the right atrium (RA) where it is mixed with poorly saturated blood from the superior vena cava (SVC). Most, however, flows directly into the left atrium (LA) through the foramen ovale and is then distributed to the brain and heart. Some of the right heart blood enters the lung, but most of it bypasses the lung through the ductus arteriosus (DA) to supply the rest of the body. Note that the net result of this somewhat complicated arrangement is that the best oxygenated blood reaches the brain and heart, and that the non-gas-exchanging lungs receive only about 15% of the cardiac output. The arterial P_{O_2} in the descending aorta is only about 22 mm Hg.

The First Breath

The emergence of the baby into the outside world is perhaps the most cataclysmic event of his or her life. He is suddenly bombarded with a variety of external stimuli. In addition, the process of birth interferes with placental gas exchange with resulting hypoxemia and hypercapnia. Finally, the sensitivity of the chemoreceptors apparently increases dramatically at birth, although the mechanism is unknown. As a consequence of all these changes, the baby makes his first gasp.

The fetal lung is not collapsed but is inflated with liquid to about 40% of total lung capacity. This fluid is continuously secreted by alveolar cells during fetal life and has a low pH. Some of it is squeezed out as the infant moves through the birth canal, but the remainder has an important role in the subsequent inflation of the lung. As air enters the lung, large surface tension forces have to be overcome. Since the larger the radius of curvature, the lower the forces (Figure 7.4), this preinflation reduces the pressures required. Nevertheless, the intrapleural pressure during the first breath may fall to −40 cm water before any air enters the lung (Figure 9.6), and peak pressures as low as −100 cm water during the first few breaths have been recorded. These very large transient pressure are partly caused by the high viscosity of the lung liquid compared with air. The fetus makes very small, rapid breathing movements in the uterus over a considerable period before birth.

Expansion of the lung is very uneven at first. However, pulmonary surfactant which is formed relatively late in fetal life is available to stabilize open alveoli, and the lung liquid is removed by the lymphatics and capillaries. Within a few moments the functional re-

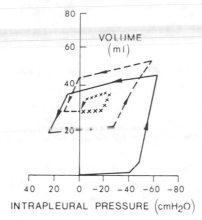

Figure 9.6. Typical intrapleural pressures developed in a newborn human infant during the first three breaths after birth. (From ME Avery: *The Lung and Its Disorders in the Newborn Infant*. Philadelphia, WB Saunders, 1968, p 29.)

sidual capacity has almost reached its normal value and an adequate gas exchanging surface has been established. However, it is several days before uniform ventilation is achieved.

Circulatory Changes

A dramatic fall in pulmonary vascular resistance follows the first few breaths. In the fetus, the pulmonary arteries are exposed to the full systemic blood pressure via the ductus arteriosus, and their walls are consequently very muscular. As a result the resistance of the pulmonary circulation is exquisitely sensitive to vasoconstrictor agents such as hypoxemia, acidosis, and serotonin, and to vasodilators such as acetylcholine. Several factors account for the fall in pulmonary vascular resistance at birth, including the abrupt rise in alveolar P_{O_2} which abolishes the hypoxic vasoconstriction, and the increased volume of the lung which widens the caliber of the extra-alveolar vessels (Figure 4.2).

With the resulting increase in pulmonary blood flow, left atrial pressure rises and the flap-like foramen ovale quickly closes. This is helped by the fall in right atrial pressure as the umbilical flow ceases. The ductus arteriosus constricts a few minutes later in response to the direct action of the increased P_{O_2} on its smooth muscle. In addition, this constriction is aided by alterations in the levels of local and circulating prostaglandins. Flow through the ductus arteriosus soon reverses as the resistance of the pulmonary circulation falls.

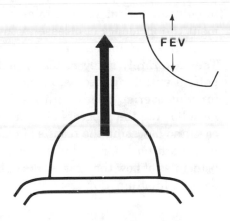

chapter **10**

Tests of Pulmonary Function

*how respiratory physiology is
applied to measure lung function**

An important practical application of respiratory physiology is the testing of pulmonary function. These tests are useful in a variety of settings. The most important is the hospital pulmonary function laboratory or, on a smaller scale, the physician's office, where these tests help in the diagnosis and the management of patients with pulmonary or cardiac diseases. In addition, they may be valuable in deciding whether a patient is fit enough for surgery. Another use is the evaluation of disability for the purposes of insurance and workman's compensation. Again, some of the simpler tests are employed

---

*This chapter is only a brief introduction to pulmonary function tests. A more detailed description can be found in JB West: *Pulmonary Pathophysiology—the essentials,* ed 3. Baltimore, Williams & Wilkins, 1987.

in epidemiological surveys to assess industrial hazards or to document the incidence of disease in the community.

The role of pulmonary function tests should be kept in perspective. They are rarely a key factor in making a definitive diagnosis in a patient with lung disease. Rather, the various patterns of impaired function overlap disease entities. While the tests are often valuable for following the progress of a patient with chronic pulmonary disease and assessing the results of treatment, in general it is far more important for the medical student (or physician) to understand the principles of how the lung works (Chapters 1–9) than to concentrate only on lung function tests.

VENTILATION

Forced Expiration

A very useful simple test of pulmonary function is the measurement of a single forced expiration. Figure 10.1 shows the spirometer record obtained when a subject inspires maximally and then exhales as hard and as completely as he can. The volume exhaled in the first second is called the forced expiratory volume, or $FEV_{1.0}$, and the total volume exhaled is the forced vital capacity, or FVC (this is often slightly less than the vital capacity measured on a slow exhalation as in figure 2.2). Normally the $FEV_{1.0}$ is about 80% of the FVC.

In disease, two general patterns can be distinguished. In *restrictive* diseases such as pulmonary fibrosis, both FEV and FVC are reduced, but characteristically the $FEV_{1.0}$/FVC% is normal or increased. In

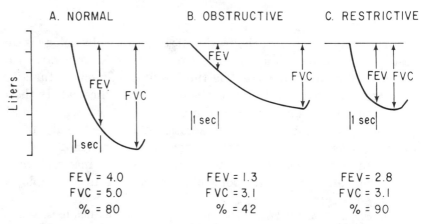

Figure 10.1. Measurement of forced expiratory volume ($FEV_{1.0}$) and forced vital capacity (FVC).

obstructive diseases such as bronchial asthma, the $FEV_{1.0}$ is reduced much more than the FVC, giving a low FEV/FVC%. Frequently mixed restrictive and obstructive patterns are seen.

A related measurement is the *forced expiratory flow rate*, or $FEF_{25-75\%}$, which is the average flow rate measured over the middle half of the expiration. Generally this is closely related to the $FEV_{1.0}$, although occasionally it is reduced when the $FEV_{1.0}$ is normal. Sometimes other indices are also measured from the forced expiration curve.

A useful way of looking at forced expirations is with *flow-volume curves,* as introduced on p. 107. Figure 10.2 reminds us that after a relatively small amount of gas has been exhaled, flow is limited by airway compression and is determined by the elastic recoil force of the lung and the resistance of the airways upstream of the collapse point. In *restrictive* diseases, the maximum flow rate is reduced, as is the total volume exhaled. However, if flow is related to the absolute lung volume (that is, including the residual volume which cannot be measured from a single expiration), the flow rate is often abnormally high during the latter part of expiration because of the increased lung recoil (Figure 10.2*B*). By contrast, in *obstructive* diseases the flow rate is very low in relation to lung volume, and a scooped-out appearance is often seen following the point of maximum flow.

What is the significance of these measurements of forced expirations? The vital capacity may be reduced at its top or bottom end (Figure 10.2). In *restrictive* diseases, inspiration is limited by the reduced compliance of the lung or chest wall, or weakness of the inspiratory muscles. In *obstructive* disease, the total lung capacity is

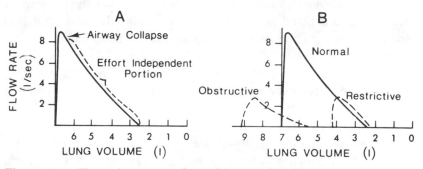

Figure 10.2. Flow volume curve obtained by recording flow rate against volume during a forced expiration from maximum inspiration. The figure shows absolute lung volumes, although these cannot be measured from single expirations.

typically abnormally large, but expiration ends prematurely. The reason for this is early airway closure brought about by increased smooth muscle tone of the bronchi as in asthma, or loss of radial traction from surrounding parenchyma, as in emphysema. Other cases include edema of the bronchial walls, or secretions within the airways.

The $FEV_{1.0}$ (or $FEF_{25-75\%}$) is reduced by an increase in airway resistance or a reduction in elastic recoil of the lung. It is remarkably independent of expiratory effort. The reason for this is the dynamic compression of airways which was discussed earlier (Figure 7.18). This mechanism explains why the flow rate is independent of the resistance of the airways downstream of the collapse point, but is determined by the elastic recoil pressure of the lung and the resistance of the airways upstream of the collapse point. The location of the collapse point is in the large airways, at least initially. Thus, both the increase in airway resistance and the reduction of lung elastic recoil pressure can be important factors in the reduction of the $FEV_{1.0}$, as for example in pulmonary emphysema.

Lung Volumes

The determination of lung volumes by spirometry and the measurement of functional residual capacity (FRC) by helium dilution and body plethysmography were discussed earlier (Figures 2.2–2.4). The FRC can also be found by having the subject breathe 100% O_2 for several minutes and washing all the N_2 out of his lung.

Suppose that the lung volume is V_1, and that the total volume of gas exhaled over 7 minutes is V_2 and that its concentration of N_2 is C_2. We know that the concentration of N_2 in the lung before washout was 80%, and we can measure the concentration left in the lung by sampling end-expired gas with an N_2 meter at the lips. Call this concentration C_3. Then, assuming no net change in the amount of N_2, we can write $V_1 \times 80 = (V_1 \times C_3) + (V_2 \times C_2)$. Thus, V_1 can be derived. A disadvantage of this method is that the concentration of nitrogen in the gas collected over 7 minutes is very low, and a small error in its measurement leads to a larger error in calculated lung volume. In addition, some of the N_2 that is washed out comes from body tissues, which should be allowed for. This method, like the helium dilution technique, measures only ventilated lung volume, whereas, as we saw on p. 14, the body plethysmograph method includes gas trapped behind closed airways.

The measurement of anatomical dead space by Fowler's method was described earlier (Figure 2.6).

DIFFUSION

The principles of the measurement of the diffusing capacity for carbon monoxide by the single breath and steady state methods were discussed on p. 27. The diffusing capacity for O_2 is very difficult to measure, and it is only done as a research procedure.

BLOOD FLOW

The measurement of total pulmonary blood flow by the Fick principle and indicator dilution were alluded to on pp. 38–39. In addition, the method of determining instantaneous pulmonary capillary flow by plethysmography was also discussed there (Figure 4.7).

VENTILATION-PERFUSION RELATIONSHIPS

Topographical Distribution of Ventilation and Perfusion

Regional differences of ventilation and blood flow can be measured using radioactive xenon as brief described earlier (Figures 2.7 and 4.8).

Inequality of Ventilation

This can be measured by single breath and multiple breath methods. The *single breath method* is very similar to that described by Fowler for measuring anatomical dead space (Figure 2.6). There we saw that if the N_2 concentration at the lips is measured following a single breath of O_2, the N_2 concentration of the expired alveolar gas is almost uniform, giving a flat "alveolar plateau." This reflects the uniform dilution of the alveolar gas by the inspired O_2. By contrast, in patients with lung disease, the alveolar N_2 concentration continues to rise during expiration. This reflects the uneven dilution of the alveolar N_2 by inspired O_2.

The reason why the concentration rises is that the poorly ventilated alveoli (those in which the N_2 has been diluted least) always empty last, presumably because they have long time constants (Figures 7.19 and 10.5). In practice the change in N_2 percentage concentration between 750 and 1250 ml of expired volume is often used as an index of uneven ventilation. This is a simple, quick, and useful test.

The *multiple breath method* is based on the rate of washout of N_2 as shown in Figure 10.3. The subject is connected to a source of 100% O_2 and a fast responding N_2 meter samples gas at the lips. If the ventilation of the lung were uniform, the N_2 concentration would be reduced by the same *fraction* with each breath. For example, if the tidal volume (excluding dead space) were equal to the FRC, the N_2 concentration would halve with each breath. In general the N_2 concentration is $FRC/[FRC + (V_T - V_D)]$ times that of the previous breath, where V_T and V_D are the tidal volume and anatomic dead space, respectively. Since the N_2 is reduced by the same fraction with each breath, the plot of log N_2 concentration against breath number would be a straight line (Figure 10.3) if the lung behaved as a single, uniformly ventilated compartment. This is very nearly the case in normal subjects.

In patients with lung disease, however, the nonuniform ventilation results in a curved plot because different lung units have their N_2 diluted at different rates. Thus, fast ventilated alveoli cause a rapid initial fall in N_2, whereas slowly ventilated spaces are responsible for the long tail of the washout (Figure 10.3).

There are various ways of expressing the inequality of ventilation from these washout curves. It is possible to describe the curves as if they were produced by two or three compartments, each having a specific ventilation rate. Such an "as if" analysis does not mean that the lung really consists of such as few homogeneous compartments,

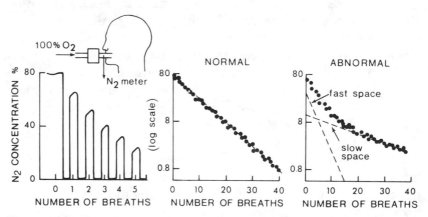

Figure 10.3. N_2 washout obtained when a subject breathes 100% O_2. Normal lungs give an almost linear plot of N_2 concentration against number of breaths on semilogarithmic paper, but this plot is nonlinear when uneven ventilation is present.

but in practice this is a convenient model for describing the amount of uneven ventilation.

Inequality of Ventilation-Perfusion Ratios

One way of assessing the mismatch of ventilation and blood flow within the diseased lung is that introduced by Riley. This is based on measurements of P_{O_2} and P_{CO_2} in arterial blood and expired gas, and the principles were briefly described at the end of Chapter 5. In practice, expired gas and arterial blood are collected simultaneously from the patient, and various indices of ventilation-perfusion inequality are computed.

One useful measurement is the *alveolar-arterial* P_{O_2} *difference*. We saw in Figure 5.11 how this develops because of regional differences in normal lung. Figure 10.4 is an O_2-CO_2 diagram which allows us to examine this development more closely. First suppose that there is no ventilation-perfusion inequality and that all the lung units are represented by a single point (i) on the ventilation-perfusion line. This is known as the "ideal" point. Now as ventilation-perfusion inequality develops, the lung units begin to spread away from i toward both $\bar{v}$ (low ventilation-perfusion ratios) and I (high ventilation-perfusion ratios) (compare Figure 5.7). When this happens, the mixed capillary blood (a) and mixed alveolar gas (A) also diverge from i. They do so along lines i to $\bar{v}$, and i to I which represent a constant respiratory exchange ratio (CO_2 output/O_2 uptake), since this is determined by the metabolism of the body tissues.[†]

The horizontal distance between A and a represents the (mixed) alveolar-arterial O_2 difference., In practice, this can only be measured easily if ventilation is essentially uniform but blood flow is uneven because only then can a representative sample of mixed alveolar gas be obtained. This is sometimes the case in pulmonary embolism. More frequently the P_{O_2} difference between ideal alveolar gas and arterial blood is calculated—the *(ideal) alveolar-arterial O_2 difference*. The ideal alveolar P_{O_2} can be calculated from the alveolar gas equation which relates the P_{CO_2} of any lung unit to the composition of the inspired gas, the respiratory exchange ratio, and the P_{CO_2} of the unit (see p. 54). In the case of ideal alveoli, the P_{CO_2} is taken to be the same as arterial blood since the line along which

---

[†] In this necessarily simplified description, some details are omitted. For example, the mixed venous point alters when ventilation-perfusion inequality develops.

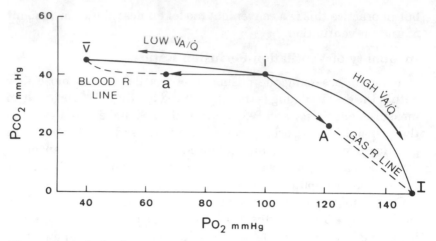

Figure 10.4. O_2-Co_2 diagram showing the ideal point i, that is, the hypothetical composition of alveolar gas and end-capillary blood when no ventilation-perfusion inequality is present. As inequality develops, the arterial (a) and alveolar (A) points diverge along their respective R (respiratory exchange ratio) lines. The mixed alveolar-arterial P_{O_2} difference is the horizontal distance between the points.

point i moves is so nearly horizontal. Note that this alveolar-arterial P_{O_2} difference is caused by units between i and $\bar{v}$, that is, those with low ventilation-perfusion ratios.

Two more indices of ventilation-perfusion inequality are frequently employed. One is *physiologic shunt* (also called *venous admixture or wasted blood flow*). For this we pretend that all of the leftward movement of the arterial point (a) away from the ideal point (i) (that is, the hypoxemia) is caused by the addition of mixed venous blood ($\bar{v}$) to ideal blood (i). This is not so fanciful as it first seems since units with very low ventilation-perfusion ratios put out blood that has essentially the same composition as mixed venous blood (Figures 5.6 and 5.7). In practice, the shunt equation (Figure 5.3) is used in the following form

$$\frac{\dot{Q}_{PS}}{\dot{Q}_T} = \frac{Ci_{O_2} - Ca_{O_2}}{Ci_{O_2} - C\bar{v}_{O_2}}$$

where $\dot{Q}_{PS}/\dot{Q}_T$ refers to the ratio of the physiological shunt to total flow. The O_2 concentration of ideal blood is calculated from the ideal P_{O_2} and O_2 dissociation curve.

The other index is *alveolar dead space*. Here we pretend that all of the movement of the alveolar point (A) away from the ideal point (i) is caused by the addition of inspired gas (I) to ideal gas. Again, this is not such an outrageous notion as it may first appear because units with very high ventilation-perfusion ratios behave very much like point I. After all, a unit with an infinitely high ventilation-perfusion ratio contains gas which has the same composition as inspired air (Figures 5.6 and 5.7). The Bohr equation for dead space (see p. 18) is used in the following form

$$\frac{V_{D_{alv}}}{V_T} = \frac{Pi_{CO_2} - PA_{CO_2}}{Pi_{CO_2}}$$

where A refers to expired alveolar gas. The result is called *alveolar dead space* to distinguish it from the *anatomic dead space*, that is, the volume of the conducting airways. Because expired alveolar gas is often difficult to collect without contamination by the anatomic dead space, the mixed expired CO_2 is often measured. The result is called the *physiologic dead space*, which includes components from the alveolar dead space *and* anatomic dead space. Since the ideal P_{CO_2} is very close to that of arterial blood (Figure 10.4), the equation for physiologic dead space is

$$\frac{V_{D_{phys}}}{V_T} = \frac{Pa_{CO_2} - PE_{CO_2}}{Pa_{CO_2}}$$

The normal value for physiologic dead space is about 30% of the tidal volume at rest and less on exercise, and it consists almost completely of anatomic dead space. In lung disease it may increase to 50% or more due to the presence of ventilation-perfusion inequality.

BLOOD GASES AND pH

P_{O_2}, P_{CO_2}, and pH are easily measured in blood samples with blood gas electrodes. A glass electrode is used to measure the pH of whole blood. The P_{CO_2} electrode is in effect a tiny pH meter in which a bicarbonate buffer solution is separated from the blood sample by a thin membrane. When carbon dioxide diffuses across the membrane from the blood, the pH of the buffer changes in accordance with the Henderson-Hasselbalch relationship. The pH meter then reads out the P_{CO_2}. The O_2 electrode is a polarograph, that is, a device which, when supplied with a suitable voltage, gives a minute current which is proportional to the amount of dissolved O_2. In practice all three electrodes are arranged to give their outputs on the same meter by appropriate switching, and a complete analysis on a blood sample can be done in a few minutes.

We saw in Chapter 5 that there are four causes of low arterial P_{O_2} or hypoxemia: (1) hypoventilation, (2) diffusion impairment, (3) shunt, and (4) ventilation-perfusion inequality.

In distinguishing between these causes it should be remembered that hypoventilation is *always* associated with a raised arterial P_{CO_2}, and that only when a shunt is present does the arterial P_{O_2} fail to rise to the expected level when 100% O_2 is administered. In diseased lungs, impaired diffusion is always accompanied by ventilation-perfusion inequality and, indeed, it is usually impossible to determine how much of the hypoxemia is attributable to defective diffusion.

There are two causes of high arterial P_{CO_2} or hypercarbia: (1) hypoventilation, and (2) ventilation-perfusion inequality. The latter does not *always* cause CO_2 retention because any tendency for the arterial P_{CO_2} to rise signals the respiratory center via the chemoreceptors to increase ventilation and thus hold the P_{CO_2} down. However, in the absence of this increased ventilation, the P_{CO_2} must rise.

The assessment of the acid-base status of the blood was discussed on pp. 77–84.

MECHANICS OF BREATHING

Lung Compliance

Compliance is defined as the volume change per unit of pressure change across the lung. In order to obtain this, we need to know intrapleural pressure. In practice, esophageal pressure is measured by having the subject swallow a small balloon on the end of a catheter. Esophageal pressure is not identical to intrapleural pressure but reflects its pressure changes fairly well. The measurement is not reliable in supine subjects because of interference by the weight of the mediastinal structures.

A simple way of measuring compliance is to have the subject breathe out from total lung capacity into a spirometer in steps of, say, 500 ml and measure his esophageal pressure simultaneously. The glottis should be open, and the lung should be allowed to stabilize for a few seconds after each step. In this way a pressure-volume curve similar to the upper line in Figure 7.3 is obtained. The whole curve is the most informative way of reporting the elastic behavior of the lung. Indices of the shape of the curve can be derived. Notice that the compliance, which is the slope of the curve, will vary depending on what lung volume is used. It is conventional to report the slope over the liter above FRC measured during deflation. Even so, the measurement is not very repeatable.

Lung compliance can also be measured during resting breathing as shown in Figure 7.13. Here we make use of the fact that at no-flow points (end of inspiration or expiration), the intrapleural pressure reflects only the elastic recoil forces and not those associated with airflow. Thus the volume difference divided by the pressure difference at these points is the compliance.

This method is not valid in patients with airway disease because the variation in time constants throughout the lung means that flow still exists within the lung when it has ceased at the mouth. Figure 10.5 shows that if we consider a lung region which has a partially obstructed airway, it will always lag behind the rest of the lung (compare Figure 7.19). In fact, it may continue to fill when the rest of the lung has begun to empty, with the result that gas moves into it from adjoining lung units—so called *pendelluft*. As the breathing

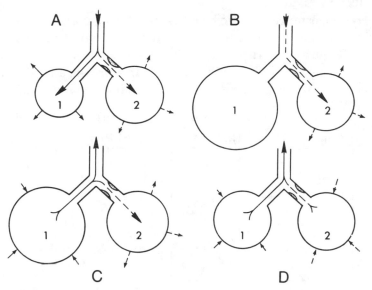

Figure 10.5. Effects of uneven time constants on ventilation. *Compartment 2* has a partially obstructed airway and, therefore, a long time constant (compare Figure 7.19). During inspiration (*A*) gas is slow to enter it, and it therefore continues to fill after the rest of the lung (*1*) has stopped moving (*B*). Indeed at the beginning of the expiration (*C*), the abnormal region (*2*) may still be inhaling while the rest of the lung has begun to exhale. In *D*, both regions are exhaling but *Compartment 2* lags behind *Compartment 1*. At higher frequencies the tidal volume to the abnormal region becomes progressively smaller.

frequency is increased, the proportion of the tidal volume that goes to this partially obstructed region becomes smaller and smaller. Thus, less and less of the lung is participating in the tidal volume changes and therefore the lung appears to become less compliant.

Airway Resistance

This is the pressure difference between the alveoli and the mouth per unit of airflow (Figure 7.12). It can be measured in a body plethysmograph (Figure 10.6).

Before inspiration (*A*), the box pressure is atmospheric. At the onset of inspiration, the pressure in the alveoli falls as the alveolar gas expands by a volume ΔV. This compresses the gas in the box and from its change in pressure ΔV can be calculated (compare Figure 2.4). If lung volume is known, ΔV can be converted into alveolar pressure using Boyle's law. Flow is measured simultaneously, and thus airway resistance is obtained. The measurement is made during expiration in the same way. Lung volume is determined as described in Figure 2.4.

Airway resistance can also be measured during normal breathing from an intrapleural pressure record as obtained with an esophageal balloon (Figure 7.13). However, in this case tissue viscous resistance is included as well (see p. 112). Intrapleural pressure reflects two sets of forces, those opposing the elastic recoil of the lung and those

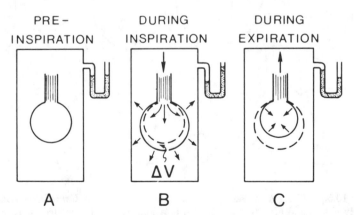

Figure 10.6. Measurement of airway resistance with the body plethysmograph. During inspiration, the alveolar gas is expanded, and box pressure therefore rises. From this, alveolar pressure can be calculated. The difference between alveolar and mouth pressure, divided by flow, gives airway resistance (see text). (Modified from J Comroe: *The Lung: Clinical Physiology and Pulmonary Function Tests,* ed 2. Chicago, Year Book, 1965, p 1979.)

overcoming resistance to air and tissue flow. It is possible to subtract the pressure caused by the recoil forces during quiet breathing because this is proportional to lung volume (if compliance is constant). The subtraction is done with an electrical circuit. We are then left with a plot of pressure against flow which gives (airway + tissue) resistance. This method is not satisfactory in lungs with severe airway disease because the uneven time constants prevent all regions from moving together (Figure 10.5).

Dynamic Compliance

We saw on p. 157 that the measurement of compliance from the intrapleural pressure at points of no flow during quiet breathing is unsatisfactory in lungs with airway disease because of uneven time constants (Figure 10.5). This apparent or "dynamic" compliance becomes smaller as the breathing frequency increases and the time for inspiration lessens, because the regions which are slow to fill receive less and less of the tidal volume. In effect an increasingly small volume of the lung participates in each breath.

It is possible to exploit this apparent limitation and use this frequency dependence of dynamic compliance as a sensitive test of increased airway resistance. We saw in Figure 7.14 that very little of the resistance of the normal bronchial tree is located in the small peripheral airways. This region, therefore, constitutes a "silent zone" in which considerable disease can occur without being detectable by measurements of total airway resistance. However, changes of resistance in peripheral airways do cause uneven time constants and therefore a change in dynamic compliance with breathing frequency. In practice, the dynamic compliance is measured at a series of frequencies from about 10 up to 120 breaths/min.

Closing Volume

Another method for detecting early disease in small airways is to use the single breath N_2 washout referred to on pp. 18 and 151, and exploit the topographical differences of ventilation discussed on p. 97 (Figures 7.8 and 7.9). Suppose a subject takes a vital capacity breath of 100% O_2 and during the subsequent exhalation the N_2 concentration at the lips is measured (Figure 10.7). Four phases can be recognized.

First, pure dead space is exhaled (1) followed by a mixture of dead space and alveolar gas (2), and then pure alveolar gas (3) (compare

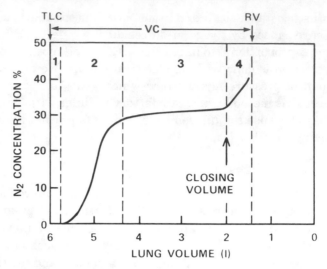

Figure 10.7. Measurement of the closing volume. If a vital capacity inspiration of 100% O_2 is followed by a full expiration, four phases in the N_2 concentration measured at the lips can be recognized (see text). The last is caused by preferential emptying of the apex of the lung after the lower zone airways have closed.

Figure 2.6). Toward the end of expiration, an abrupt increase in N_2 concentration is seen (4). This signals closure of airways at the base of the lung (Figure 7.9) and is caused by preferential emptying of the apex, which has a relatively high concentration of N_2. The reason for the higher N_2 at the apex is that during a vital capacity breath of O_2, this region expands less (Figure 7.9) and, therefore, the N_2 there is less diluted with O_2. Thus, the volume of the lung at which dependent airways begin to close can be read off the tracing.

In young normal subjects, the closing volume is about 10% of the vital capacity (VC). It increases steadily with age and is equal to about 40% of the VC, that is the FRC, at about the age of 65 years. Relatively small amounts of disease in the small airways apparently increase the closing volume, although the mechanism of this is not yet fully understood.

CONTROL OF VENTILATION

The responsiveness of the chemoreceptors and respiratory center to CO_2 can be measured by having the subject rebreathe into a rubber bag as discussed on p. 124. We saw that the alveolar P_{O_2} also affects ventilation so that if the response to CO_2 alone is required, the inspired P_{CO_2} should be kept above 200 mm Hg to avoid any hypoxic drive. The ventilatory response to hypoxia can be measured in a similar way if the subject rebreathes from a bag with a low P_{O_2} but constant P_{CO_2}.

EXERCISE

Additional information about pulmonary function can often be obtained if tests are made when the subject exercises. The resting lung has enormous reserves; its ventilation, blood flow, O_2 and CO_2 transfer, and diffusing capacity can be increased several-fold on exercise. Frequently, patients with early disease have pulmonary function tests that are within normal limits at rest, but abnormalities are revealed when the respiratory system is stressed by exercise.

Methods of providing controlled exercise include the treadmill and bicycle ergometer. Measurements most often made on exercise include total ventilation, pulse rate, O_2 uptake, CO_2 output, respiratory exchange ratio, arterial blood gases, and the diffusing capacity of the lung for carbon monoxide.

PERSPECTIVE ON TESTS OF PULMONARY FUNCTION

In this chapter we have touched on some of the lung function tests that are presently available. In conclusion it should be emphasized that not all these tests are commonly used in a hospital pulmonary function laboratory. Only a few can be used in a doctor's office or on an epidemiological survey.

The most useful simple test in the clinical setting is the *forced expiration*. It does not matter much which indices are derived from this test, but the $FEV_{1.0}$ and FVC are very frequently reported. Next, the ability to measure *arterial blood gases* is essential if patients with respiratory failure are managed and is valuable in any case. After these, the relative importance of tests becomes more a matter of personal preference, but a well-equipped pulmonary function laboratory would be able to measure lung volumes, inequality of ventilation, alveolar-arterial P_{O_2} difference, physiologic dead space and shunt, diffusing capacity for carbon monoxide, airway resistance, lung compliance, ventilatory response to CO_2 and hypoxia, and the patient's response to exercise. In large laboratories, more specialized measurements such as the topographical distribution of ventilation and blood flow would be available.

Appendix

SYMBOLS

Primary

C   Concentration of gas in blood
F   Fractional concentration in dry gas
P   Pressure or partial pressure
Q   Volume of blood
$\dot{Q}$ Volume of blood per unit time
R   Respiratory exchange ratio
S   Saturation of hemoglobin with O_2
V   Volume of gas
$\dot{V}$ Volume of gas per unit time

Secondary Symbols for Gas Phase

A   Alveolar
B   Barometric
D   Dead space
E   Expired
I   Inspired
L   Lung
T   Tidal

Secondary Symbols for Blood Phase

a   arterial
c   capillary
c'   end-capillary
i   ideal
v   venous
$\bar{v}$ mixed venous

Examples

O_2 concentration in arterial blood Ca_{O_2}
Fractional concentration N_2 in expired gas FE_{N_2}
Partial pressure of O_2 in mixed venous blood $P\bar{v}_{O_2}$

UNITS

Traditional metric units have been used in this book. Pressures are given in mm Hg; the torr is an almost identical unit.

In Europe, SI (Système Internationale) units are now commonly used. Most of these are familiar, but the kilopascal, the unit of pressure, is confusing at first. One kilopascal = 7.5 mm Hg (approximately).

EQUATIONS

Gas Laws

General gas law: $PV = RT$

where T is temperature and R is a constant. This equation is used to correct gas volumes for changes of water vapor pressure and temperature. For example, ventilation is conventionally reported at BTPS, that is, body temperature (37°C), ambient pressure, and saturated with water vapor. By contrast, gas volumes in blood are expressed as STPD, that is, standard temperature (0°C or 273°K) and pressure (760 mm Hg) and dry. To convert a gas volume at BTPS to one at STPD, multiply by

$$\frac{273}{310} \cdot \frac{P_B - 47}{760}$$

where 47 mm Hg is the water vapor pressure at 37°C.

Boyle's law	$P_1V_1 = P_2V_2$	(temperature constant)
and *Charles' law*	$\dfrac{V_1}{V_2} = \dfrac{T_1}{T_2}$	(pressure constant)

are special cases of the general gas law.

Avogadro's law states that equal volumes of different gases at the same temperature and pressure contain the same number of molecules. A gram molecule, for example, 32 gm of O_2, occupies 22.4 liters at STPD.

Dalton's law states that the partial pressure of a gas (x) in a gas mixture is the pressure that this gas would exert if it occupied the total volume of the mixture in the absence of the other components.

Thus, $P_x = P \cdot F_x$, where P is the total dry gas pressure since F_x conventionally refers to dry gas. In gas with a water vapor pressure of 47 mm Hg

$$P_x = (P_B - 47) \cdot F_x$$

Also, in the alveoli, $P_{O_2} + P_{CO_2} + P_{N_2} + P_{H_2O} = P_B$.

The *partial pressure of a gas in solution* is its partial pressure in a gas mixture which is in equilibrium with the solution.

Henry's law states that the concentration of gas dissolved in a liquid is proportional to its partial pressure. Thus, $C_x = K \cdot P_x$.

Ventilation

$$V_T = V_D + V_A$$

where V_A here refers to the volume of alveolar gas in the tidal volume.

$$\dot{V}_A = \dot{V}_E - \dot{V}_D$$

$$\dot{V}_{CO_2} = \dot{V}_A \cdot F_{A_{CO_2}} \qquad \text{(both } \dot{V} \text{ measured at BTPS)}$$

$$\dot{V}_A = \frac{\dot{V}_{CO_2}}{P_{A_{CO_2}}} \times K \qquad \text{(alveolar ventilation equation)}$$

If $\dot{V}_A$ is BTPS and $\dot{V}_{CO_2}$ is STPD, $K = 0.863$. In normal subjects $P_{A_{CO_2}}$ is nearly identical to $P_{a_{CO_2}}$.

Bohr equation

$$\frac{V_D}{V_T} = \frac{P_{A_{CO_2}} - P_{E_{CO_2}}}{P_{A_{CO_2}}}$$

Or, using arterial P_{CO_2}

$$\frac{V_D}{V_T} = \frac{P_{a_{CO_2}} - P_{E_{CO_2}}}{P_{a_{CO_2}}}$$

This gives *physiologic dead space*.

Diffusion

In the *gas phase, Graham's law* states that the rate of diffusion of a gas is inversely proportional to its molecular weight.

In *liquid or a tissue slice, Fick's law** states that the volume of gas per unit time which diffuses across a tissue sheet is given by

$$\dot{V}_{gas} = \frac{A}{T} \cdot D \cdot (P_1 - P_2)$$

where A and T are the area and thickness of the sheet, P_1 and P_2 are the partial pressure of the gas on the two sides, and D is a diffusion

---

*Fick's law was originally expressed in terms of concentrations, but partial pressures are more convenient for us.

constant sometimes called the permeability coefficient of the tissue for that gas.

This *diffusion constant* is related to the solubility (Sol) and the molecular weight (MW) of the gas

$$D \propto \frac{Sol}{\sqrt{MW}}$$

When the diffusing capacity of the lung (D_L) is measured with carbon monoxide and the capillary P_{CO} is taken as zero,

$$D_L = \frac{\dot{V}_{CO}}{P_{A_{CO}}}$$

D_L is made up of two components. One is the diffusing capacity of the alveolar membrane (D_M) and the other depends on the volume of capillary blood (V_c) and the rate of reaction of CO with hemoglobin θ

$$\frac{1}{D_L} = \frac{1}{D_M} + \frac{1}{\theta V_c}$$

Blood Flow

Fick principle

$$\dot{Q} = \frac{\dot{V}_{O_2}}{Ca_{O_2} - C\bar{v}_{O_2}}$$

Pulmonary vascular resistance

$$PVR = \frac{P_{art} - P_{ven}}{\dot{Q}}$$

where P_{art} and P_{ven} are the mean pulmonary arterial and venous pressures, respectively.

Starling's law of fluid exchange across the capillaries

$$\text{Net flow out} = K[(P_c - P_i) - \sigma(\pi_c - \pi_i)]$$

where i refers to the interstitial fluid around the capillary, π to the colloid osmotic pressure, and K is the filtration coefficient.

Ventilation-Perfusion Relationships

Alveolar gas equation

$$P_{A_{O_2}} = P_{I_{O_2}} - \frac{P_{A_{CO_2}}}{R} + \left[P_{A_{CO_2}} \cdot F_{I_{O_2}} \cdot \frac{1-R}{R} \right]$$

This is only valid if there is no CO_2 in inspired gas. The term in square brackets is a relatively small correction factor when air is breathed (2 mm Hg when $P_{CO_2} = 40$, $F_{IO_2} = 0.21$, and $R = 0.8$). Thus, a useful approximation is

$$PA_{O_2} = PI_{O_2} - \frac{PA_{CO_2}}{R}$$

Respiratory exchange ratio
If no CO_2 is present in the inspired gas

$$R = \frac{\dot{V}_{CO_2}}{\dot{V}_{O_2}} = \frac{PE_{CO_2}(1 - F_{IO_2})}{PI_{O_2} - PE_{O_2} - (PE_{CO_2} \cdot F_{IO_2})}$$

Venous to arterial shunt

$$\frac{\dot{Q}_s}{\dot{Q}_T} = \frac{Cc'_{O_2} - Ca_{O_2}}{Cc'_{O_2} - C\bar{v}_{O_2}}$$

where c′ means end-capillary.
Ventilation-perfusion ratio equation

$$\frac{\dot{V}_A}{\dot{Q}} = \frac{8.63 \ R(Ca_{O_2} - C\bar{v}_{O_2})}{PA_{CO_2}}$$

where blood gas concentrations are in ml/100 ml.
Physiologic shunt

$$\frac{\dot{Q}_{PS}}{\dot{Q}_T} = \frac{Ci_{O_2} - Ca_{O_2}}{Ci_{O_2} - C\bar{v}_{O_2}}$$

Alveolar dead space

$$\frac{V_D}{V_T} = \frac{Pi_{CO_2} - PA_{CO_2}}{Pi_{CO_2}}$$

The equation for *physiologic dead space* is on p. 165.

Blood Gases and pH

O_2 dissolved in blood

$$C_{O_2} = Sol \cdot P_{O_2}$$

where Sol is 0.003 ml O_2/100 ml blood/mm Hg.

Henderson-Hasselbalch equation

$$pH = pK_A + \log \frac{(HCO_3^-)}{(CO_2)}$$

The pK_A for this system is normally 6.1. If HCO_3^- and CO_2 concentrations are in millimoles per liter, CO_2 can be replaced by P_{CO_2} (mm Hg) × 0.030.

Mechanics of Breathing

Compliance = $\Delta V/\Delta P$
Specific compliance = $\Delta/V/(V \cdot \Delta P)$
Laplace equation for pressure caused by surface tension of a sphere

$$P = 2T/r$$

where r is the radius. Note that for a soap bubble, $P = 4T/r$, because there are two surfaces.

Poiseuille's law for laminar flow

$$\dot{V} = (P\pi r^4)/8nl$$

where n is the coefficient of viscosity† and P is the pressure difference across the length l.

Reynolds number

$$Re = 2rvd/n$$

where v is average linear velocity of the gas, d is its density, and n its viscosity.

Pressure drop for laminar flow, $P\alpha\dot{V}$, but for turbulent flow, $P\alpha\dot{V}^2$ (approximately).

Airway resistance

$$\frac{P_{alv} - P_{mouth}}{\dot{V}}$$

where P_{alv} and P_{mouth} refer to alveolar and mouth pressures.

---

† This is a corruption of the Greek letter η, for those of us who have little Latin and less Greek.

Questions

(for answers see p. 174–176)
Note: When several possible answers are given, more than one may be correct.

CHAPTER 1

1. What is the approximate area and thickness of the blood-gas barrier, and what are the physiological advantages of its morphology?
2. What is the P_{O_2} of moist inspired gas of a climber on the summit of Mount Everest (assume barometric pressure is 247 mm Hg)?
3. What tissue layers does oxygen pass through on its way from the alveolar gas to the interior of a red blood cell in the pulmonary capillary?
4. How is a respiratory bronchiole distinguished from a terminal bronchiole?
5. According to Weibel's idealization, how many branchings have the airways, and approximately how many of these are in the conducting zone?
6. What is the chief mechanism of gas movement in the respiratory zone?
7. Approximately how long does a red cell spend in the pulmonary capillaries, and how many alveoli does it traverse in this time?
8. How are dust particles cleared from the lung after they settle on the walls of the larger airways?

CHAPTER 2

1. Which of the following lung volumes cannot be measured with a simple spirometer: (a) vital capacity: (b) functional residual capacity; (c) tidal volume; (d) residual volume?
2. Approximately what proportion of the resting lung volume (FRC) is contained in the anatomic dead space? What happens to (a) the volume of the dead space, and (b) the proportion, when lung volume is increased to TLC?
3. In a measurement of FRC by helium dilution, the original and final helium concentrations were 10 and 6%, and the spirometer volume was kept at 5 liters. What was the volume of the FRC?
4. A subject sits in a body plethysmograph and makes an expiratory effort against his closed glottis. What happens to the pressure in the plethysmograph?
5. If alveolar ventilation doubles and CO_2 production remains constant, what happens to arterial P_{CO_2}?
6. If alveolar and mixed expired P_{CO_2} are 40 and 30 mm Hg, respectively, what is the physiologic dead space from the Bohr equation?
7. A pressure tank of dry gas at 3000 mm Hg pressure contains 80% O_2. What is the partial pressure and fractional concentration of the O_2?
8. If the total ventilation and CO_2 production remain constant, which of the following will decrease the arterial P_{CO_2} (a) increase in respiratory frequency; (b) increase in FRC; (c) increase in tidal volume; (d) increase in inspired O_2 concentration?
9. When radioactive xenon is inhaled, which region of the lung receives most of the gas: (a) upper zone; (b) lower zone?

CHAPTER 3

1. Write down Fick's law of gas diffusion as applied to a tissue slice.
2. If gas X is twice as soluble and twice as dense as gas Y, which diffuses faster in solution?

3. A subject inhales several breaths of a gas mixture containing low concentrations of carbon monoxide and nitrous oxide. For which gas will the partial pressures in arterial blood and alveolar gas be nearly identical?

4. Which of the following are most likely to result in diffusion limitation of O_2 uptake: (a) exercise; (b) breathing a high O_2 mixture; (c) thickening of alveolar wall by disease?

5. An exercising subject breathes a low concentration of CO in a steady state. If his alveolar P_{CO} is 0.5 mm Hg and his CO uptake is 30 ml/min, what is the diffusing capacity of his lung for CO? What units is it expressed in?

6. What is the relation between the diffusing capacity of the lung (D_L), diffusing capacity of the alveolar membrane (D_M), volume of the capillary blood (V_C), and rate of reaction of CO with hemoglobin θ?

7. In the uptake of O_2, is the resistance offered by diffusion across the blood-gas barrier (a) much greater than, (b) much less than, or (c) approximately equal to the resistance offered by the rate of combination of O_2 with hemoglobin?

8. Is the time taken for the P_{CO_2} of blood to reach virtually the same partial pressure as alveolar gas along the pulmonary capillary (a) much less, (b) much more, (c) about the same, as that for O_2?

CHAPTER 4

1. How much smaller is the mean pressure in the pulmonary artery, compared with that in the aorta?

2. What pressures are the pulmonary capillaries exposed to? Is the pressure surrounding a larger vessel (for example, 1 mm diameter artery) (a) less, (b) greater, (c) about the same?

3. If the mean pulmonary arterial and left atrial pressures are 20 and 8 mm Hg, respectively, and total pulmonary blood flow is 5 liters/min, what is the pulmonary vascular resistance? What are the units?

4. What are the mechanisms for the fall in pulmonary vascular resistance which occurs on exercise?

5. Why does pulmonary vascular resistance rise (a) at low lung volumes, (b) at high lung volumes (if alveolar pressure is not changed with respect to vascular pressures)?

6. Which of the following drugs injected into the pulmonary circulation typically increase pulmonary vascular resistance: (a) serotonin; (b) acetylcholine; (c) norepinephrine?

7. If the O_2 concentrations of mixed venous and arterial blood are 16 and 20 ml/100 ml, respectively, and O_2 consumption is 300 ml/min, what is the total pulmonary blood flow?

8. In the zone of the lung where alveolar pressure exceeds venous pressure, what is the pressure difference responsible for blood flow?

9. Hypoxic vasoconstriction of pulmonary blood vessels occurs (a) in response to a reduce P_{O_2} in the pulmonary arterial blood, (b) in response to a reduced P_{O_2} in the alveolar gas, (c) via a reflex arc involving the spinal cord.

10. In early pulmonary edema, fluid in seen in (a) interstitial space of alveolar wall, (b) perivascular spaces, (c) alveolar space.

11. The metabolics functions of the lung include (a) converting angiotensin I to II, (b) inactivating bradykinin, (c) liberating erythropoietin.

CHAPTER 5

1. A man with normal lungs and arterial P_{CO_2} of 40 mm Hg takes an overdose of barbiturate which halves his alveolar ventilation but does not change his CO_2 output. What will his arterial P_{CO_2} rise to? If his respiratory exchange ratio is 0.8, approximately how much will his arterial P_{O_2} fall? How much does the inspired O_2 concentration have to be raised to abolish the hypoxemia?

2. A man with normal lungs and a right-to-left shunt is found at catheterization to have O_2 concentrations in his arterial and mixed venous blood of 18 and 14 ml/100 ml, respectively. If the O_2 concentration of the blood leaving the pulmonary capillaries is calculated to be 20 ml/100 ml, how large is his shunt? Will his arterial P_{O_2} rise if he is given 100% O_2 to breathe?

3. When the ventilation-perfusion ratio of a lung unit increases, does the (a) alveolar P_{O_2} rise, (b) alveolar P_{CO_2} fall, (c) alveolar P_{N_2} remain the same?

4. Many patients with ventilation-perfusion inequality have hypoxemia but no CO_2 retention because (a) CO_2 diffuses more rapidly than O_2 (b) the O_2 and CO_2 dissociation curves have different shapes, (c) the solubility of CO_2 in blood is much higher than that of O_2.

5. The apex of the upright human lung, compared with the base, has a (a) high P_{O_2}, (b) high ventilation, (c) high pH in end-capillary blood.

6. If a lung with no uneven ventilation and blood flow suddenly develops ventilation-perfusion inequality, the immediate changes will be (a) fall in arterial P_{O_2}, (b) fall in O_2 uptake, (c) rise in arterial P_{CO_2}, (d) fall in CO_2 output.

7. A patient whose arterial P_{O_2} and P_{CO_2} are both 40 mm Hg when he is breathing air has marked ventilation-perfusion inequality but no shunt. When given 100% O_2 to breathe, his ventilation remains unchanged. His arterial P_{O_2} will probably rise to (a) above 500 mm Hg, (b) between 200 and 500 mm Hg, (c) below 200 mm Hg.

8. Physiologic dead space can be increased by (a) lung units with high ventilation-perfusion ratios, (b) unventilated lung units, (c) enlargement of anatomic dead space.

CHAPTER 6

1. A patient being treated with hyperbaric O_2 has an arterial P_{O_2} of 2000 mm Hg and his arterial-venous O_2 difference is 5 ml/100 ml. Will the hemoglobin in his mixed venous blood probably be fully saturated?

2. A man is accidentally exposed to carbon monoxide which combines with half the hemoglobin in his arterial blood. Will his (a) arterial P_{O_2}, (b) arterial O_2 content, (c) P_{O_2} in mixed venous blood be normal, high, or low?

3. Which of the following shift the O_2 dissociation curve to the left: (a) reduction in temperature, (b) reduction in pH, (c) reduction in P_{CO_2}, (d) reduction in 2,3-diphosphoglycerate in the red cell?

4. In what form is most of the CO_2 carried in the (a) arterial or (b) venous blood?

5. Carbonic anhydrase is found (a) only in the plasma, (b) only in the red cells, (c) equally in plasma and red cells.

6. When CO_2 is given off by blood in the lungs (a) chloride ions move into the red cells, (b) the loading of O_2 is assisted, (c) the red cells shrink slightly.

7. If a normal subject develops respiratory alkalosis by hyperventilation for a minute, is his arterial plasma bicarbonate concentration altered? If a diabetic patient develops metabolic acidosis without respiratory compensation, is his arterial P_{CO_2} altered?

8. A patient with chronic lung disease was found to have an arterial P_{CO_2} of 60 mm Hg and pH of 7.35. How is his acid-base status best described? After being treated by assisted ventilation for 3 days, his arterial P_{CO_2} was found to be 40 mm Hg and pH 7.32. What was his probable acid-base status then?

9. In acute carbon monoxide poisoning, is the (a) P_{O_2}, or (b) O_2 content of mixed venous blood normal, low, or high? What about acute cyanide poisoning?

CHAPTER 7

1. When the diaphragm contracts, the lateral distance between the lower margins of the ribs (a) increases, (b) decreases, or (c) remains the same.

2. Which of the following decrease pulmonary compliance: (a) increasing age, (b) alveolar edema, (c) saline inflation of the lung?

3. Two bubbles have the same surface tension, but bubble X has three times the diameter of bubble Y. What is the relationship between the pressures within the bubbles?

4. Pulmonary surfactant is formed by the (a) alveolar macrophages, (b) goblet cells, (c) Type I alveolar cells, (d) Type II alveolar cells.

5. "Interdependence" refers to (a) effect of surface tension forces on capillary pressure, (b) stabilizing forces generated by expanded alveoli on neighboring units, (c) effect of change in vascular pressures on transpulmonary pressure.

6. When a pneumothorax is induced, the chest wall (a) collapses in, (b) expands out, (c) remains where it was.

7. According to Poiseuille's law, how much will the resistance of a tube increase when its radius is reduced to one-third?

8. When a diver is at a great depth and the density of the air is increased, is turbulence more or less likely to occur in large airways?

9. During expiration, which pressure is higher (less negative)—alveolar or intrapleural? What about during inspiration?

10. During normal breathing, most of the resistance to flow is in the (a) trachea, (b) medium sized airways, (c) airways less than 2 mm in diameter.

11. Why is airway resistance decreased at high lung volumes?

12. During most of a forced expiration, flow rate is limited by (a) contraction of expiratory muscles, (b) inertia of chest wall, (c) compression of airways.

13. Two lung lobes, X and Y, have the same airway resistance, but X has three times the compliance of Y. Which will be the slower to empty during passive expiration?

14. What breathing pattern might a patient with a normal airway resistance but very stiff lungs (low compliance) adopt which would reduce his work of breathing?

CHAPTER 8

1. What pattern of breathing results if a cat brain is sectioned just above the pontine apneustic center?

2. Which of the following in arterial blood exerts the most important control on ventilation under normal conditions: (a) P_{O_2}, (b) P_{CO_2}, (c) pH?

3. Which of the following reduces the ventilatory response to inhaled CO_2: (a) obstruction to breathing, (b) alveolar hypoxia, (c) administration of morphine?

4. Do the peripheral chemoreceptors respond chiefly to the P_{O_2} in arterial or mixed venous blood? Does mild carbon monoxide poisoning increase ventilation?

5. Explain why a hypoxemic patient with chronic CO_2 retention may develop a very high arterial P_{CO_2} when given 100% O_2 to breathe.

6. The Hering-Breuer inflation reflex (a) results in further inspiratory efforts if the lung is maintained inflated, (b) is only seen in adult man at high tidal volumes, (c) may help to inflate the newborn lung.
7. Muscle spindles in the intercostal muscles may (a) play a role in the production of dyspnea, (b) help to maintain ventilation when the compliance of the lung is suddenly altered, (c) allow the ribs to rotate on the vertebrae.
8. Which of the following play a part in the increase in ventilation on moderate exercise: (a) reflexes from moving limbs, (b) increase in body temperature, (c) fall in arterial P_{O_2}, (d) rise in arterial P_{CO_2}?

CHAPTER 9

1. What is the normal pH of the CSF? What sequence of changes occurs in the CSF pH when a lowlander moves to high altitude for several days?
2. List three features of acclimatization to high altitudes which are physiologically advantageous.
3. Why is the gas in a pneumothorax gradually absorbed?
4. What are the advantages of helium-oxygen over air as a breathing mixture for very deep dives?
5. Why should an amateur scuba diver never fill his tank with 100% O_2?
6. What are three mechanisms of deposition of inhaled aerosols and how are these related to the size of the particle? How are particles which deposit in the alveoli removed?
7. Why is CO_2 retention difficult to prevent during liquid breathing?
8. What factors promote closure of the foramen ovale at birth?

CHAPTER 10

1. What is the (a) 1 second forced expiratory volume, (b) forced expiratory flow rate ($FEF_{25-75\%}$)?
2. What factors reduce the $FEV_{1.0}$ in pulmonary emphysema?
3. In the single breath test of uneven ventilation, why does the N_2 concentration in alveolar gas rise more steeply in the presence of uneven ventilation than in the normal lung?
4. How is the ideal alveolar P_{O_2} derived in a patient with lung disease?
5. List four causes of hypoxemia. Which two may cause CO_2 retention?
6. Why does dynamic compliance decrease with increase of breathing frequency in the abnormal lung?
7. Explain how the "closing volume" can be measured when a subject exhales after inspiring a vital capacity breath of O_2.

Answers

CHAPTER 1

1. 50–100 square meters; less than ½ micron in many parts; large area and small thickness are well suited to diffusion of gas.
2. Approximately 42 mm Hg.
3. Surfactant, alveolar epithelium interstitial layer, capillary endothelium, plasma, red cell interior.
4. By the alveoli budding from its walls.
5. 23, 16.
6. Gaseous diffusion.
7. ½ to 1 second, 2 to 3 alveoli (probably).
8. Transported up to the epiglottis on the layer of mucus which is moved by ciliary action, then swallowed.

CHAPTER 2

1. b, d.
2. About 5%; (a) increases, (b) decreases.
3. 3.3 liters.
4. Decreases.
5. Halves.
6. 0.25 of tidal volume.
7. 2400 mm Hg, 0.8.
8. c.
9. b.

CHAPTER 3

1. $\dot{V} \text{ gas} = \frac{A}{T} D \cdot (P_1 - P_2).$
2. X.
3. Nitrous oxide.
4. a, c.
5. 60 ml/min/mm Hg.
6. $\frac{1}{D_L} = \frac{1}{D_M} + \frac{1}{\theta \cdot V_c}$
7. c.
8. c.

CHAPTER 4

1. About six times.
2. Alveolar approximately, a.
3. 2.4 mm Hg/liter/min.
4. Recruitment and distention of blood vessels.
5. Extra-alveolar vessels narrow; capillaries narrow (probably).
6. a, c.
7. 7.5 liters/min.
8. Pulmonary arterial minus alveolar.
9. b (mainly).

10. a, b.
11. a, b.

CHAPTER 5

1. 80 mm Hg; approximately 50 mm Hg; about 7% (or 0.07).
2. One-third of total flow; yes.
3. (a) yes, (b) yes, (c) no.
4. b.
5. a, c.
6. a, b, c, d.
7. a.
8. a, c.

CHAPTER 6

1. Yes.
2. (a) normal, (b) low, (c) low.
3. a, c, d.
4. (a) bicarbonate, (b) bicarbonate.
5. b.
6. b, c.
7. Yes; no.
8. Partially compensated respiratory acidosis; metabolic acidosis.
9. For CO poisoning (a) low, (b) low; for cyanide poisoning (a) high, (b) high.

CHAPTER 7

1. a.
2. b.
3. Pressure in X is one-third of pressure in Y.
4. d.
5. b.
6. b.
7. 81 times.
8. More.
9. Alveolar; alveolar.
10. b.
11. Increased caliber of bronchi because of tethering to surrounding parenchyma.
12. c.
13. X.
14. Shallow, rapid breathing.

CHAPTER 8

1. Long inspiratory gasps.
2. b.
3. a, c.
4. Arterial; no.
5. Most of his ventilatory drive is due to his hypoxemia because the pH of his CSF has returned toward normal and his arterial blood pH is normal (or nearly so). Therefore, giving him 100% results in reduced ventilation.

6. b.
7. a, b.
8. a, b.

CHAPTER 9

1. 7.32; first CSF pH rises because the P_{CO_2} in the CSF falls; then the bicarbonate concentration falls, and the CSF pH is returned toward normal.
2. Hyperventilation, polycythemia (probably), changes in intracellular oxidative enzymes.
3. Because the sum of the partial pressures of gases in the venous blood is less than that in the pneumothorax gas.
4. Less risk of decompression sickness and inert gas narcosis; also, lower density reduces work of breathing.
5. Because of the danger of convulsions caused by O_2 toxicity on the CNS.
6. Impaction for large particles, sedimentation for medium-sized particles, diffusion for small particles; engulfed by macrophages which leave via the lymphatics and blood.
7. Because of the limited rate of diffusion of CO_2 in the airways of the respiratory zone.
8. Rise of pressure in left atrium due to increased pulmonary blood flow; fall of pressure in right atrium as umbilical flow ceases.

CHAPTER 10

1. (a) Volume exhaled in 1 second by forced expiration from total lung capacity; (b) average flow rate measured over middle half (by volume) of forced expiration.
2. Increased airway resistance and reduced static recoil forces.
3. Poorly ventilated units have a relatively high N_2 concentration, and they empty last because they have long time constants.
4. By using the alveolar gas equation with arterial P_{CO_2}.

$$P_{O_2} = PI_{O_2} - \frac{Pa_{CO_2}}{R} + [F]$$

5. Hypoventilation, ventilation-perfusion inequality, diffusion impairment , shunt, first two.
6. Because the regions with long time constants receive less and less of the tidal volume.
7. The N_2 concentration of the upper zone is high because it receives less O_2. Therefore, when lower zone airways close toward the end of expiration, a sharp increase in N_2 concentration is measured.

Further Reading

This list includes some classical papers and some more recent reviews.

Structure and Function

DEJOURS P: *Principles of Comparative Respiratory Physiology.* Amsterdam, North Holland, 1975.

HAYEK H VON: *The Human Lung,* translated by VE Krahl. New York, Hafner, 1960.

HODSON WA: *Development of the Lung.* New York, Dekker, 1977.

MURRAY JF: *The Normal Lung,* ed 2. Philadelphia, WB Saunders, 1986.

WEIBEL ER: *Morphometry of the Human Lung.* New York, Academic Press, 1963.

WEIBEL ER, TAYLOR CR: Design and structure of the human lung. In Fishman AP (ed): *Pulmonary Diseases and Disorders,* ed 2. New York, McGraw Hill, 1988.

Ventilation

BOUHUYS A, LUNDIN G: Distribution of inspired gas in lungs. *Physiol Rev* 39:731–750, 1959.

CUMMING G, CRANK J, HORSFIELD K, PARKER I: Gaseous diffusion in the airways of the human lung. *Respir Physiol* 1:58–74, 1966.

ENGEL LA, PAIVA M: *Gas Mixing and Distribution in the Lung.* New York, Dekker 1985.

FOWLER WS: Intrapulmonary distribution of inspired gas. *Physiol Rev* 32:1–20, 1952.

OTIS AB, MCKERROW CB, BARTLETT RA, MEAD J, MCILROY MB, SELVERSTONE NJ, RADFORD EP: Mechanical factors in distribution of pulmonary ventilation. *J Appl Physiol* 8:427–443. 1956.

Diffusion

FORSTER RE: Diffusion of gases across the alveolar membrane. In Farhi L, Tenney SM: *Handbook of Physiology. The Respiratory System.* Bethesda, MD, American Physiological Society, 1987, vol 4, sect 3, pp 71–88.

KROGH M: The diffusion of gases through the lungs of man. *J Physiol (Lond)* 49:271–300, 1914–1915.

OGILVIE CM, FORSTER RE, BLAKEMORE WS, MORTON JW: A standardized breath-holding technique for the clinical measurement of the diffusing capacity of the lung for carbon monoxide. *J Clin Invest* 36:1–17, 1957.

ROUGHTON FJW, FORSTER RE: Relative importance of diffusion and chemical reaction rates in determining rate of exchange of gases in the human lung, with special reference to true diffusing capacity of pulmonary membrane and volume of blood in the lung capillaries. *J Appl Physiol* 11:290–302, 1957.

WAGNER PD: Diffusion and chemical reaction in pulmonary gas exchange. *Physiol Rev* 57:257–312, 1977.

Blood Flow and Metabolism

BAKHLE YS, VANE JR (eds): *Metabolic Functions of the Lung.* New York, Dekker, 1977.

FUNG YC, SOBIN SS: Theory of sheet flow in lung alveoli. *J Appl Physiol* 26:472–488, 1969.

GLAZIER JB, HUGHES JMB, MALONEY JE, WEST JB: Measurements of capillary dimensions and blood volume in rapidly frozen lungs. *J Appl Physiol* 26:65–76, 1969.

HARRIS P, HEATH D: *The Human Pulmonary Circulation,* ed 2. Edinburgh and London, Livingstone, 1978.

LEE G, DUBOIS AB: Pulmonary capillary blood flow in man. *J Clin Invest* 34:1380–1390, 1955.

PERMUTT S, RILEY RL: Hemodynamics of collapsible vessels with tone: the vascular waterfall. *J Appl Physiol* 18:924–932, 1963.

WEST JB, DOLLERY CT, NAIMARK A: Distribution of blood flow in isolated lung: relation to vascular and alveolar pressures. *J Appl Physiol* 19:713–724, 1964.

Ventilation-Perfusion Relationships

RAHN H, FENN WO: *A Graphical Analysis of the Respiratory Gas Exchange. The O_2-CO_2 Diagram.* Washington, DC, American Physiological Society, 1955.

RILEY RL, COURNAND A: 'Ideal' alveolar air and the analysis of ventilation-perfusion relationships in the lungs. *J Appl Physiol* 1:825–847, 1949.

RILEY RL, COURNAND A: Analysis of factors affecting partial pressures of oxygen and carbon dioxide in gas and blood of lungs: theory. *J Appl Physiol* 4:77–101, 1951.

WEST JB: *Ventilation/Blood Flow and Gas Exchange,* ed 4. Oxford, Blackwell, 1985.

West JB: State of the art: ventilation-perfusion relationships. *Am Rev Respir Dis* 116:919–943, 1977

Gas Transport to the Periphery

ASTRUP P: A new approach to acid-base metabolism. *Clin Chem* 7:1–15, 1961.

BAUMANN R: Blood oxygen transport. In Farhi L, Tenney SM: *Handbook of Physiology. The Respiratory System.* Bethesda, MD, American Physiological Society, 1987, vol 4, sect 3, pp 147–172.

DAVENPORT HW: *The ABC of Acid Base Chemistry,* ed 6. Chicago, University of Chicago Press, 1974.

KLOCKE RA: Carbon dioxide transport. In Farhi L, Tenney SM: *Handbook of Physiology. The Respiratory System.* Bethesda, MD, American Physiology Society, 1987, vol 4, sect 3, pp 173–198.

ROUGHTON FJW: Transport of oxygen and carbon dioxide. In Fenn WO, Rahn H: *Handbook of Physiology. Respiration.* Washington, DC, American Physiological Society, 1964, vol 1, sect 3, pp 767–826.

SEVERINGHAUS JW: Electrodes for blood and gas P_{CO_2}, P_{O_2} and blood pH. *Acta Anesthesiol Scand* (Suppl.) 11:207–220, 1962.

Mechanics of Breathing

CAMPBELL EJM, AGOSTONI E, DAVID JN: *The Respiratory Muscles: Mechanics and Neural Control,* ed 2. Philadelphia, WB Saunders, 1970.

HOPPIN FG, HILDEBRANDT J: Mechanical properties of the lung. In West JB: *Bioengineering Aspects of the Lung.* New York, Dekker, 1977.

MACKLEM PT: Airway obstruction and collateral ventilation. *Physiol Rev* 51:368–436, 1971.

MILIC-EMILI J, HENDERSON JAM, DOLOVICH MB, TROP D, KANEKO K: Regional distribution of inspired gas in the lung. *J Appl Physiol* 21:749–759, 1966.

PEDLEY TJ, SCHROTER RC, SUDLOW MF: Gas flow and mixing in airways. In West JB: *Bioengineering Aspects of the Lung.* New York, Dekker, 1977.

PRIDE NB, PERMUTT S, RILEY RL, BROMBERGER-BARNEA B: Determinants of maximum expiratory flow from the lungs. *J Appl Physiol* 23:646–662, 1967.

RAHN H, OTIS AB, CHADWICK LE, FENN WO: The pressure-volume diagram of the thoiax and lung: Am J Physiol 146.161=116, 1946.

Control of Ventilation

BERGER AJ, MITCHELL RA, SEVERINGHAUS JW: Regulation of respiration. *N Engl J Med* 297:92–97, 138–143, 194–201, 1977.
CHERNIACK RM, SNIDAL DP: The effect of obstruction to breathing on the ventilatory response to CO_2. *J Clin Invest* 35:1286–1290, 1956.
CUNNINGHAM DJC, LLOYD BB (eds): *The Regulation of Human Respiration*. Oxford, Blackwell, 1963.
GUYTON AC, CROWELL JW, MOORE JW: Basic oscillating mechanism of Cheyne-Stokes breathing. *Am J Physiol* 187:395–398, 1956.
HORNBEIN TF: *Regulation of Breathing*. New York, Dekker, 1981.
HOWELL JBL, CAMPBELL EJM: *Breathlessness*. Philadelphia, Davis, 1966.
PORTER R (ed): *Hering-Breuer Centenary Symposium*. Ciba Foundation Symposium. London, Churchill, 1970.
VON EULER C: On the central pattern generator for the basic breathing rhythmicity. *J Appl Physiol Respirat Environ Exercise Physiol* 55:1647–1659, 1983.

Respiratory Physiology Function in Unusual Environments

BARCROFT J: *The Respiratory Function of the Blood. Part I. Lessons from High Altitude*. London, Cambridge University Press, 1925.
BERT P: *Barometric Pressure. Researches in Experimental Physiology,* translated by MA Hitchcock and FA Hitchcock. Columbus, Ohio, College Book Co., 1943.
DAWES GS: *Foetal and Neonatal Physiology: A Comparative Study of the Changes at Birth*. Chicago, Year Book, 1968.
HURTADO A: Animals in high altitudes: resident man. In Dill DB: *Handbook of Physiology, Adaptation to the Environment*. Washington, DC, American Physiological Society, 1964, sect 4, pp 843–860.
LAMBERTSEN CJ (ed): Underwater physiology. In: *Proceedings of the Fourth Symposium on Underwater Physiology*. New York, Academic Press, 1971.
STRAUSS RH: *Diving Medicine*. New York, Grune & Stratton, 1976.
WARD MP, MILLEDGE JS, WEST JB: *High Altitude Medicine and Physiology*. London, Chapman and Hall; Philadelphia, University of Pennsylvania Press, 1989.
WEST JB, LAHIRI S: *High Altitude and Man*. Washington, DC, American Physiological Society, 1984.

Tests of Pulmonary Function

BATES DV, MACKLEM PT, CHRISTIE RV: *Respiratory Function in Disease,* ed 2. Philadelphia, WB Saunders, 1971.
CHERNIACK RM, CHERNIACK L, NAIMARK A: *Respiration in Health and Disease,* ed 2. Philadelphia, WB Saunders, 1972.
COTES JE: *Lung Function: Assessment and Application in Medicine,* ed 4. Oxford, Blackwell, 1979.
FORSTER RE, FISHER AB, DUBOIS AB, BRISCOE WA: *Physiological Basis of Pulmonary Function Tests,* ed 3. Chicago, Year Book, 1986.
WEST JB: *Pulmonary Pathophysiology—the essentials,* ed 3. Baltimore, Williams & Wilkins, 1987.

Index

181